Cardiac Rhythm Management - Pacing, Ablation, Devices

Edited by Mart Min and Gabriel Cismaru

Published in London, United Kingdom

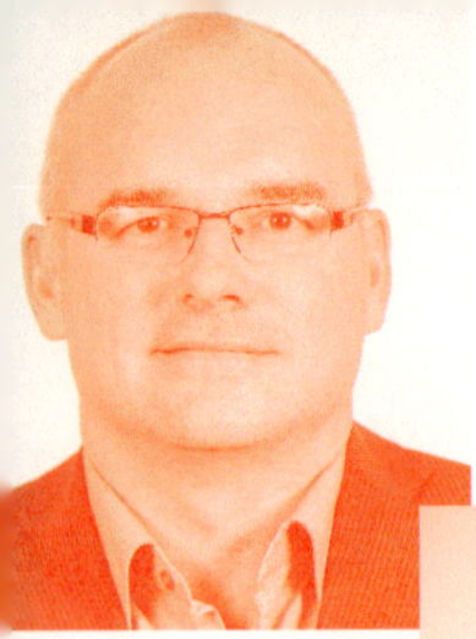
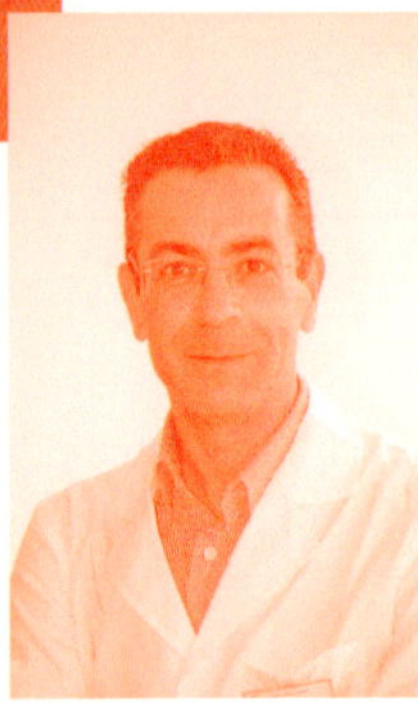
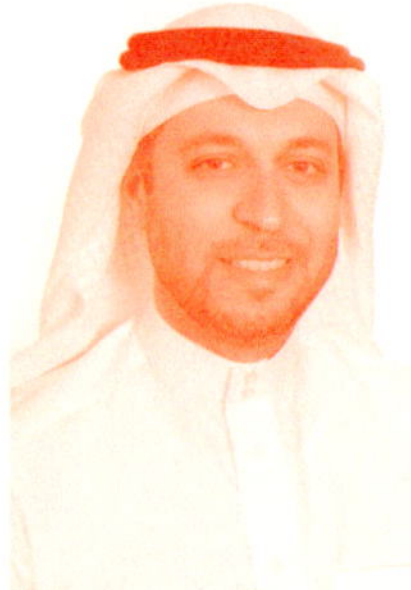
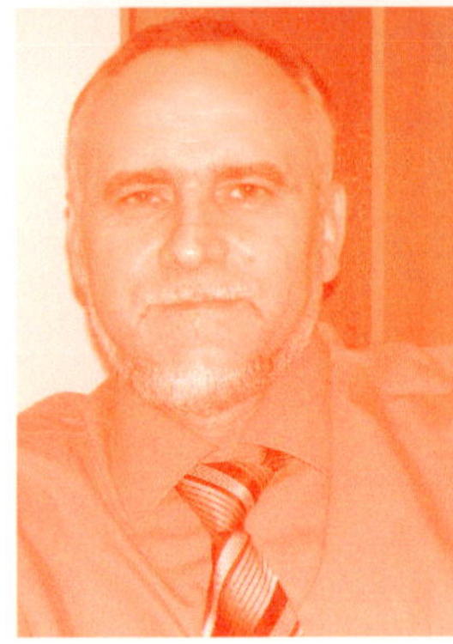
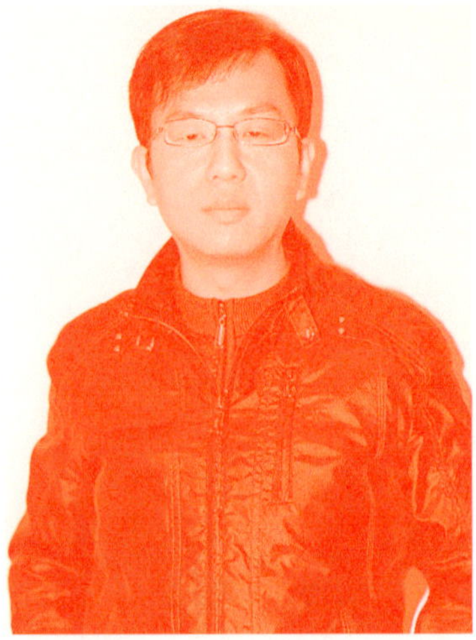
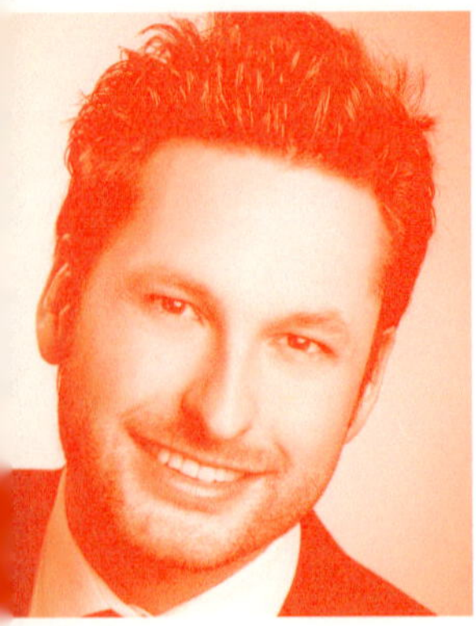
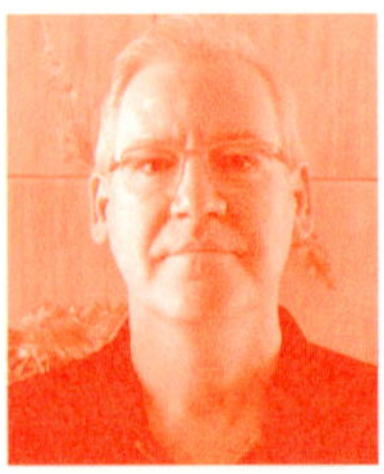

IntechOpen

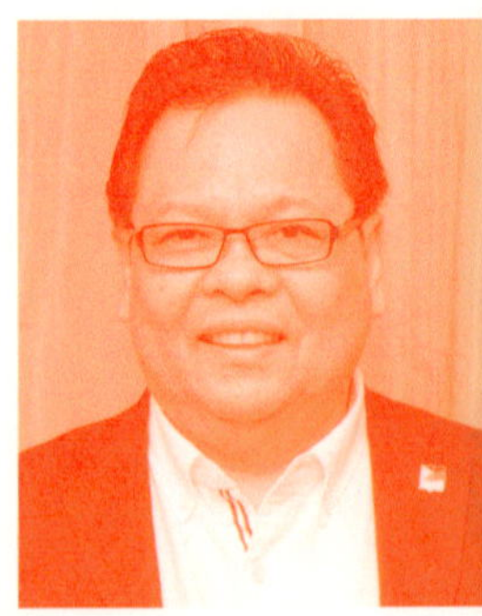
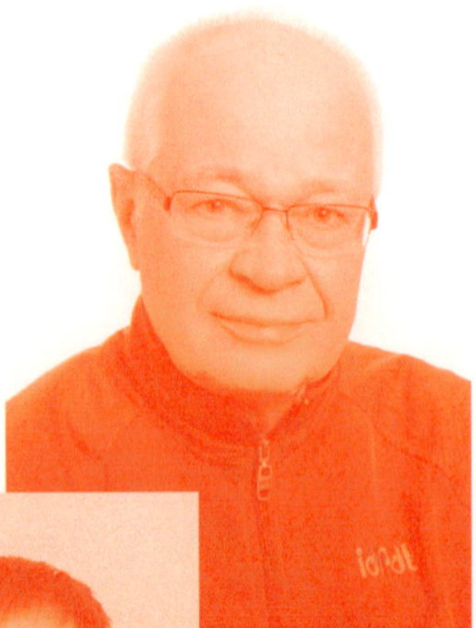
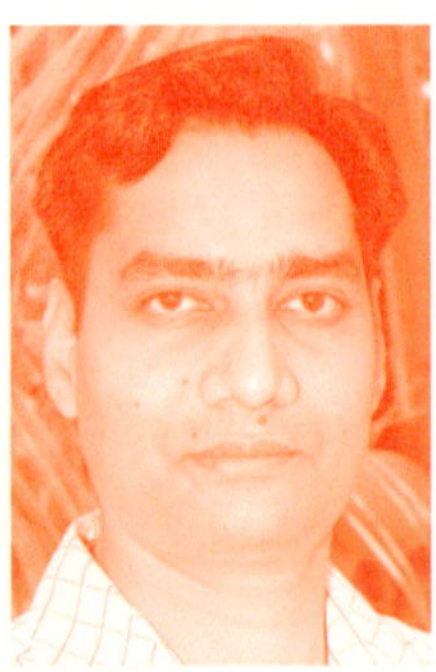
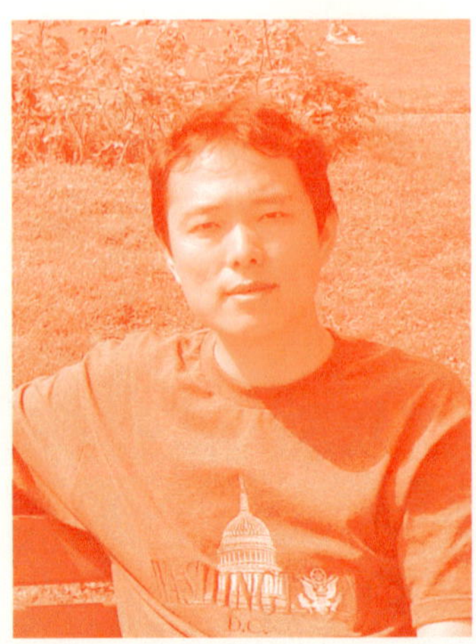
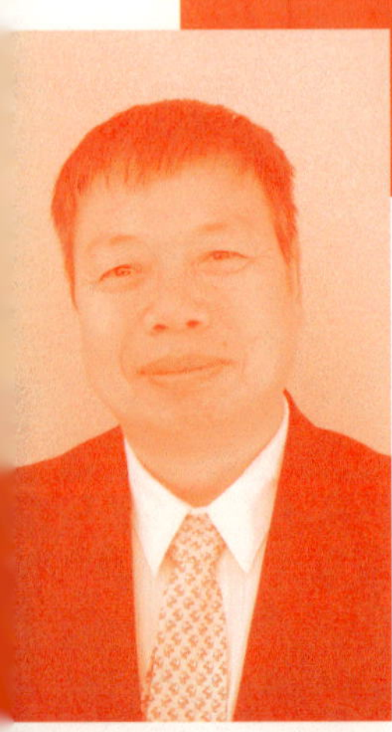
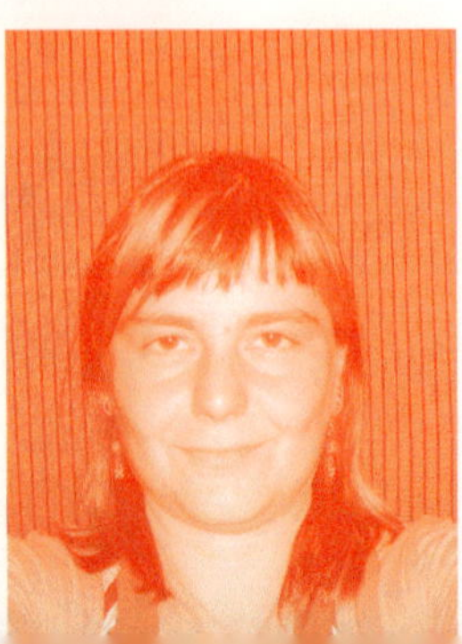

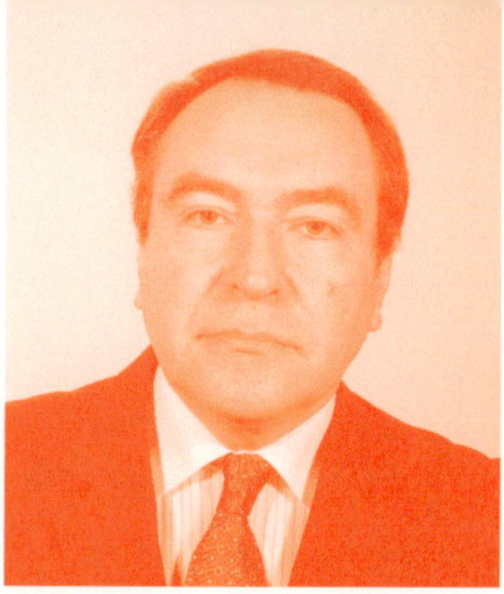
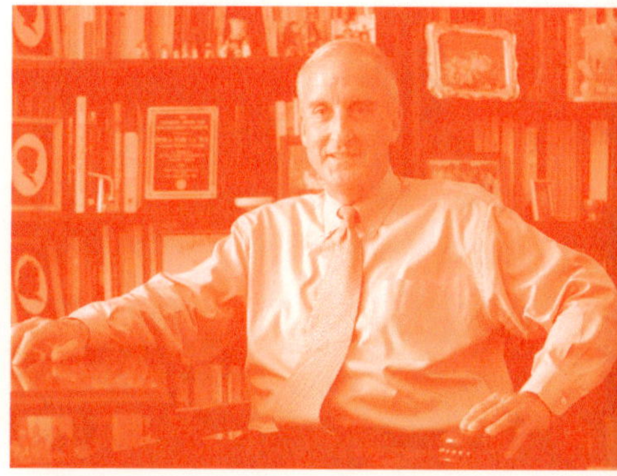
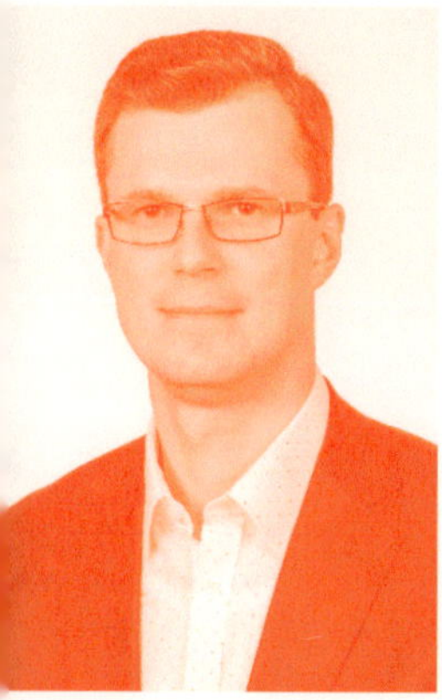
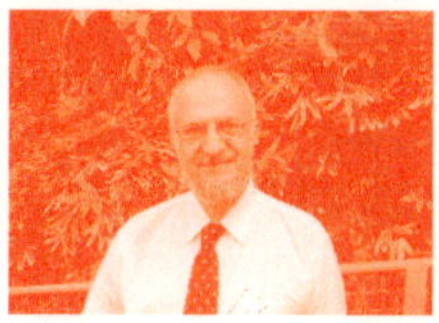
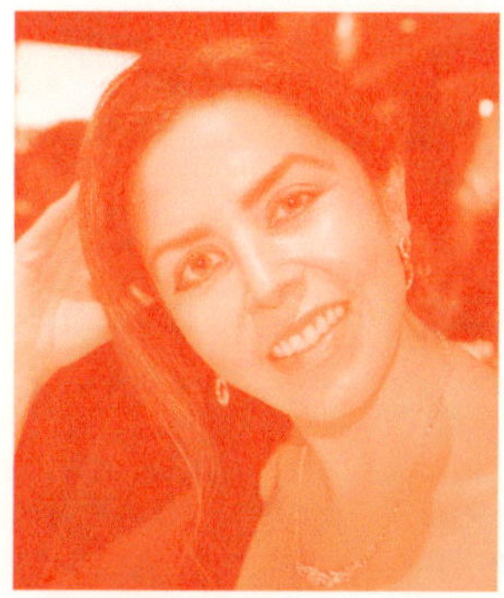

Supporting open minds since 2005

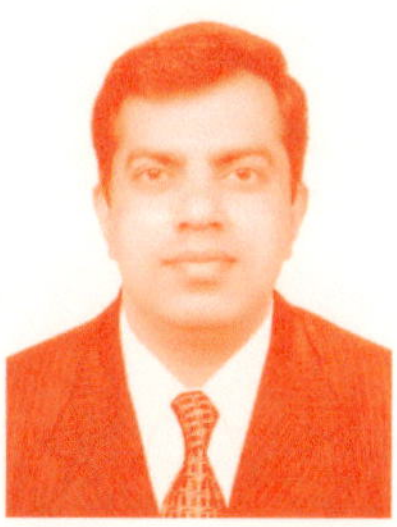
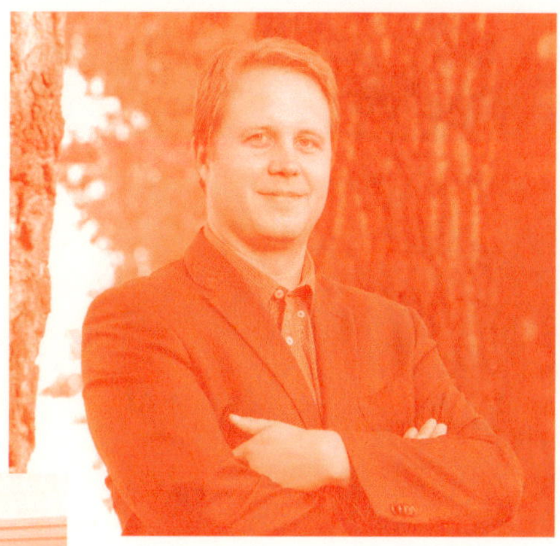
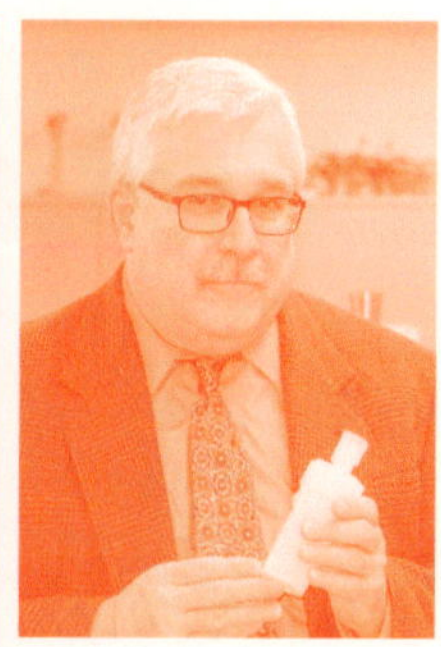
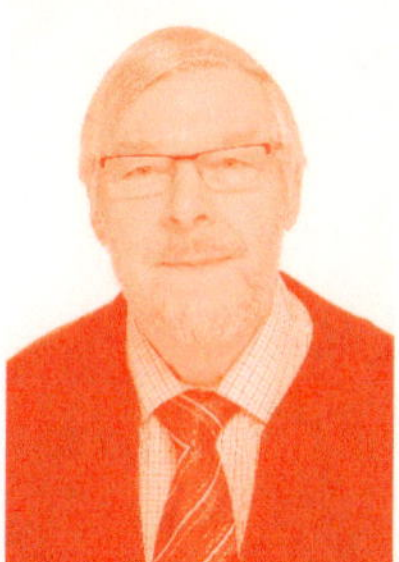
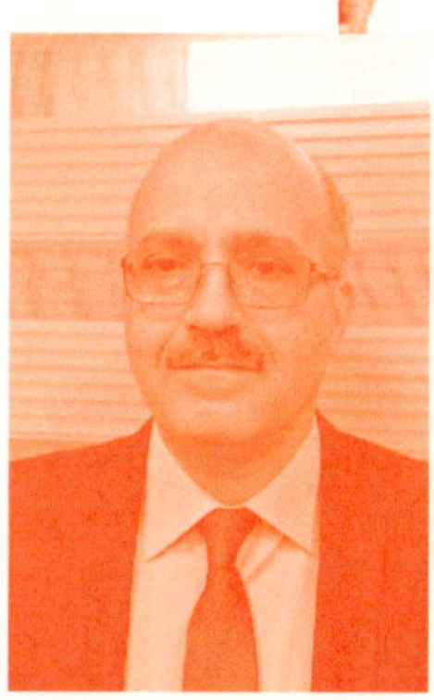
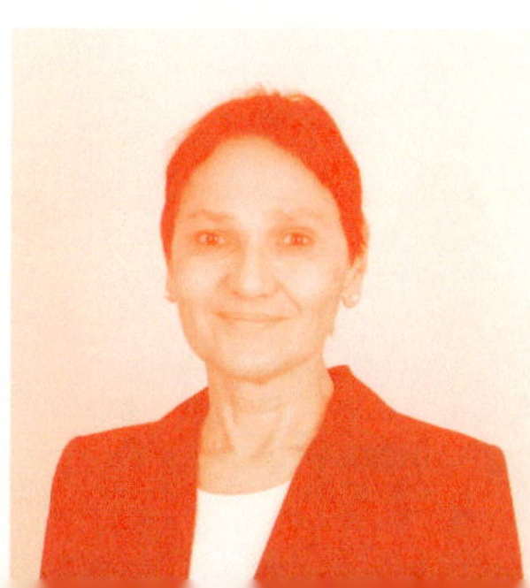
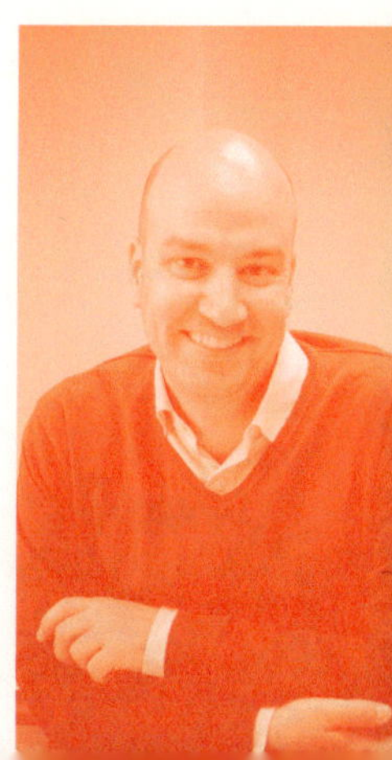

Cardiac Rhythm Management - Pacing, Ablation, Devices
http://dx.doi.org/10.5772/intechopen.95171
Edited by Mart Min and Gabriel Cismaru

Assistant to the Editors: Raluca Tomoaia

Contributors
Chin-Yu Lin, Kamran Ghods, Shahrzad Aghaamoo, Narges Amini, Hoda Zangian, Mohamad Foroozesh, Jo Ann LeQuang, Joseph V. Pergolizzi, Peter Magnusson, Nándor Szegedi, László A Gellér, Abdullah Alabdulgader, Jacek Kot, Mart Min, Gabriel Cismaru

First published in London, United Kingdom, 2022 by IntechOpen
IntechOpen is the global imprint of INTECHOPEN LIMITED, registered in England and Wales, registration number: 11086078, 5 Princes Gate Court, London, SW7 2QJ, United Kingdom
Printed in Croatia

British Library Cataloguing-in-Publication Data
A catalogue record for this book is available from the British Library

Additional hard and PDF copies can be obtained from orders@intechopen.com

Cardiac Rhythm Management - Pacing, Ablation, Devices
Edited by Mart Min and Gabriel Cismaru
p. cm.
Print ISBN 978-1-80355-009-1
Online ISBN 978-1-80355-010-7
eBook (PDF) ISBN 978-1-80355-011-4

For EU product safety concerns:
IN TECH d.o.o., Prolaz Marije Krucifikse Kozulić 3, 51000 Rijeka, Croatia, info@intechopen.com or visit our website at intechopen.com.

Meet the editors

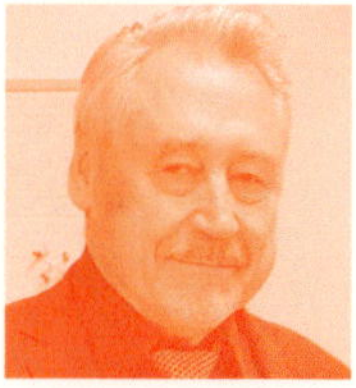

Mart Min is a full professor and leading scientist at the Thomas Johann Seebeck Department of Electronics, Tallinn University of Technology, Estonia. He received a Diploma Engineer's qualification in Electronics from the same university in 1969, and a Ph.D. in Measurement Science from Kyiv Polytechnic, Ukraine in 1984. From 1992 to 1993 he was a guest scientist and professor at the Technical University of Munich and Bundeswehr University, Germany. From 2007 to 2010 he was a leading scientist at the international research group of the Institute of Bioprocessing and Analytical Measurement Technique, Germany. Dr. Min is interested in electronic measurements and signal processing methods with implementations in medicine, including the development of rate-responsive cardiac pacemakers for US companies. He is an author and co-author of more than 250 papers and 40 patents as well as an editor of several scientific books in biomedical engineering. He is a senior life member of the Institute of Electrical and Electronics Engineers (IEEE) Instrumentation and Measurement Society and Engineering in Medicine and Biology Society. He is a member of the International Committee for Promotion of Research in Bio-Impedance (ICPRBI). Professor Emeritus since 2017, Dr. Min continues activities as a research scientist in biomedical electronics.

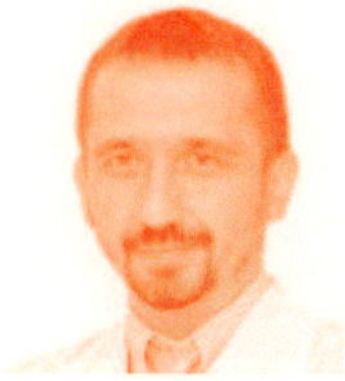

Dr. Cismaru Gabriel is an assistant professor at the Cluj-Napoca University of Medicine and Pharmacy, Romania, where he has been qualified in cardiology since 2011. He obtained his Ph.D. in medicine with a research thesis on electrophysiology and pro-arrhythmic drugs in 2016. Dr. Cismaru began his electrophysiology fellowship at the Institut Lorrain du Coeur et des Vaisseaux Louis Mathieu, France, after finishing his cardiology certification with stages in Clermont-Ferrand and Dinan, France. He began working at the Rehabilitation Hospital's Electrophysiology Laboratory in Cluj-Napoca in 2011. He is an experienced operator who can implant pacemakers, CRTs, and ICDs, as well as perform catheter ablation of supraventricular and ventricular arrhythmias such as ventricular tachycardia and ventricular fibrillation. He has been qualified in pediatric cardiology since 2022, and he regularly performs device implantation and catheter ablation in children. Dr. Cismaru has authored or co-authored peer-reviewed publications and book chapters on cardiac pacing, defibrillation, electrophysiological studies, and catheter ablation.

Contents

Preface

Cardiovascular disease (CVD) is currently known to be one of the leading causes of death in the world. The World Health Organization (WHO) reported that CVD is responsible for one-third of all deaths globally. The annual cost of CVD to the world economy is estimated to be more than a trillion US dollars. The prevalence of CVD raises an urgent need to improve patient outcomes.

A significant proportion of CVD is associated with heart rhythm problems, which means that the rhythm responds poorly or not at all to the physiological needs of the body. There is both an excessively slow rhythm (bradycardia) and an excessively high rhythm (tachycardia) or an unstable rhythm (arrhythmia, rhythm disturbances). Fortunately, many methods, techniques, and tools have been developed and successfully applied today to stabilize and control heart rate. These measures benefit many millions of people every year.

Not only electrical pacing but also ablation is an effective minimally invasive surgical method and technique to reduce and block arrhythmias, both as an independent treatment method or in conjunction with pacing therapy. Radiofrequency ablation (RFA) has revolutionized the treatment of both supraventricular and ventricular arrhythmias. The development of novel mapping systems has led to the ablation of more complex arrhythmias such as atrial tachycardia, atrial fibrillation (AF), and ventricular tachycardia (VT).

This book reviews modern cardiac rhythm management methods and devices together with some important medical aspects of their use. Written by the editors, Chapter 1 provides a developmental insight into modern methods and devices for cardiac rhythm management, both for electrical pacing and radio frequency ablation. Chapter 2 addresses the implantation problems of different pacing devices, focusing on both the surgical side and postoperative care. Chapter 3 discusses the possibilities of using pacemakers in under-water conditions. Chapter 4 examines the nature of pain after the insertion of implantable devices and how to reduce it. Chapter 5 looks at the past, present, and future directions in the development of cardiac resynchronization therapy (CRT). Chapters 6 and 7 discuss the problems of ablation, highlighting the short but strong pulse method and RFA of the epicardium.

The editors believe that the dedicated work of authors will provide readers with theoretical knowledge and practical guidance as well as the tools and skills to overcome the problems of heart rate management in their professional activities.

Mart Min
Tallinn University of Technology,
Tallinn, Estonia

Gabriel Cismaru
Iuliu Hațieganu University of Medicine and Pharmacy,
Cluj-Napoca, Romania

Chapter 1

Introductory Chapter: Modern Methods and Devices for Cardiac Rhythm Management

Mart Min and Gabriel Cismaru

1. Introduction

Cardiovascular disease (CVD), which refers to interdependently related heart and blood vessel problems, is currently known to be one of the leading causes of death in the world. The World Health Organization (WHO) reported that CVD is responsible for one-third of all deaths globally. The annual cost of CVD to the economy is estimated about £25 billion in the UK and over $500 billion in the USA. The prevalence and cost of CVD raise an urgent need for solutions to elevate standards of care and improve patient outcomes.

A significant proportion of CVD is associated with heart rhythm problems, which means that the rhythm responds poorly or not at all to the physiological needs of the body. There are both an excessively slow rhythm (bradycardia) and an excessively high rhythm (tachycardia) or an unstable rhythm (arrhythmia, rhythm disturbances). All these incorrect rhythm phenomena are life-threatening. Fortunately, many methods, techniques, and tools have been developed and successfully applied today to stabilize and control the heart rate (HR). Modern implantable devices and treatment methods, including minimally invasive surgery, have been developed for cardiac rhythm management and avoiding heart failure. These measures benefit many millions of people every year [1].

Not only electrical pacing [1–3], but also ablation is an effective minimally invasive surgical method for reducing and blocking arrhythmic phenomena [4, 5], both as an independent treatment method and in conjunction with pacing therapy. In the following, we will look at modern cardiac rhythm management methods and devices in more detail together with some important medical aspects of their use.

2. Making the devices smarter

2.1 Historical glimpse

The implementation of artificial pacing goes back more than 70 years [6]. The first electrical devices connected to a patient to provide electrical impulses to stimulate the heartbeat in bradycardia cases have been known since the 1950s. Thanks to the invention of silicon transistor in 1956, the 1958 was a remarkable milestone. In winter 1958, engineer Earl Bakken of Minneapolis, USA, co-founder of Medtronic company, produced the first wearable external pacemaker for a patient of C. Walton Lillehei. On October 8, 1958, the first electronic pacemaker was implanted by Senning and Elmqvist in Solna, Sweden. In 1958, Dr. William Chardack teamed up with engineer Wilson Greatbatch and Dr. Andrew Gage to implant an electrode in a dog attached to a pulse generator. They worked for the next two years to refine their design of a unit. They implanted the pacemaker into a man and commercialized the product in 1960.

All the early pacemakers maintain the same constant pulse rhythm for long periods of time. A pacemaker in demand also appeared in the 1960s, which only paced when stimulation was required (when natural pacing ceased). In addition, the dual-chamber pacemaker with synchronized pacing of both atrium and ventricle (known as physiological pacing) was first designed in 1960s [6]. In the end of this period are included also first attempts to use the variable pacing rhythm to adapt it to a physiological need, i.e., the metabolic requirement corresponding to body's work known as rate-responsive pacing [7]. The medical use of rate-responsive pacing began in early 1980s [8].

2.2 Sensing and sensors for the adaptive and closed-loop control of pacing rate

The problem is: how to get information for the adjusting of pacing rate? Obviously, it is almost impossible to use the body's natural sensing nodes for this purpose; the help of artificial means or sensors is required [7, 8]. Some of the proposed information sources for regulating the pacing rate are oxygen saturation level, venous pH, QT interval, activity of body motions, respiratory rate, minute volume (MV), stroke volume (SV), central venous temperature, peak endocardial acceleration, and electrical impedance changes of the right ventricle (reflects a stroke volume) during the whole cardiac cycle. QT interval (reflecting both physiological and mental status) and minute volume (MV) sensors based on the electrical bioimpedance measurement of a tidal volume (TV) of lungs and stroke volume (SV) and cardiac output (CO) sensors based on the measurement of the internal bioimpedance of the left ventricle have been lifted onto the shield. There is no single sensor giving adequate information for regulating the pacing rate. The carefully weighted resultant from multiple sensors can provide reliable information for setting the pacing rate. Artificial intelligence methods, the results of which are under strict supervisory inspection to avoid the possibility of fatal error, can be the direction for future developments [9–11].

2.3 Principles of bioimpedance sensing

For bioimpedance sensing, a low-level microamp (μA) range alternating current (AC) excitation of kilohertz range (kHz) is delivered from one electrode to another, and the caused voltage drop is measured. For example, these electrodes can be the pacing electrodes inside the right ventricle (in apex) and the case of implanted pacemaker [9]. Between these electrodes are situating both breathing lungs and contracting/relaxing myocardium of the beating heart [9–13]. As a result, we can measure the dynamic impedance of breathing lungs $Z_L(t)$ and of working myocardium $Z_M(t)$. The impedance $Z_L(t)$ gives the bases for calculating the tidal volume (TV), respiration rate (RR), and minute volume $MV = TV \times RR$ in liters. It is well known how the minute volume (MV) of breathing correlates with the physical work W of patient's organism, which, in turn, determines the need for a fresh oxygen-rich blood expressed through a stroke volume (SV) and cardiac output $CO = SV \times HR$ in liters. Heart rate (HR) is equal to pacing rate (PR) for pacemaker patients. Therefore, the pacing rate (PR) determines the amount of oxygen-rich blood (CO) directly. The described mechanism forms the pacing rate (PR) management principle in modern cardiac rhythm devices. However, because we do not know exactly the functional relationship between the required blood volume (CO) and PR, it becomes necessary to measure the effective CO and compare it with the desired comparison and negative feedback. With this, we achieve the automatic PR adjustment based on the feedback principle of closed-loop control [8, 14]. The feedback mechanism is provided determining the resulting stroke volume (SV) and cardiac output (CO) via measuring the electrical bioimpedance Z_V of the right ventricle, which is inversely proportional to stroke volume [13].

2.4 Supervisory control of pacing rate limits

For the benefit of the patient, it is reasonable not to rigidly fix the upper and lower pacing rate limits, but to leave them sliding within certain limits depending on the patient's current medical condition. At the same time, however, both underpacing and overpacing must be strictly avoided. Both are dangerous for life, especially overpacing that can cause myocardial infarction, and must be strictly avoided [13, 14]. The principle is that the body demand for oxygen-rich blood must not exceed the ability of patient's injured heart. Energy balance between the energy supply and energy consumption of myocardium must be fulfilled in every moment of heart work. The balance conditions and overpacing risk were derived from the measurement of myocardial impedance Z_M [12]. Underpacing risk was derived from the bioimpedance Z_V measurement of ventricular volume—too large volumes indicate underpacing danger for the myocardium [12, 13].

2.5 Traditional and novel methods for delivering the pacing pulses

2.5.1 Traditional single-chamber pacing

The most known location of the pacing electrode is the tip (apex cavity) of the right ventricle. This solution has been working well for many decades in cardiac pacemakers to prevent bradycardia since the invention of the portable/wearable pacemaker in the 1950s and the widespread use of the implantable device in the 1960s [6]. In addition, the most modern leadless pacemakers [15] use only the ventricular pacing. Many implantable cardioverter defibrillators (ICDs) use only the ventricular pacing to restore unstable or failed heart rate to its normal beating through timed electrical shock delivery.

2.5.2 Dual-chamber pacing

Later, in the mid-1970s, a dual-chamber pacing—one pacing electrode in the ventricular apex and another in the atrium of heart's right side—has been introduced in medical practice [6]. The dual-chamber pacing most closely resembles the normal physiology of cardiac initiation, compared to other pacemaker modes. Therefore, this device is also called as a physiological pacemaker, which ensures atrium-ventricle timing (synchronization) and suppresses atrial fibrillation (AF), that is, reduces the risk of pacemaker syndrome, which represents the clinical consequences of atrioventricular dyssynchrony after pacemaker implantation. Dual-chamber implantable cardioverter defibrillators (ICDs) provide dual-chamber pacing to prevent both atrial fibrillation and supraventricular tachycardia not available in single-chamber ICDs [16]. Nowadays, most of the currently implanted ICD devices provide overdrive pacing to convert ventricular tachycardia (VT) or deliver electrical shocks to restore normal rhythm in the case of sustained ventricular tachycardia or ventricular fibrillation.

2.5.3 Biventricular pacing

Biventricular pacing, also called as cardiac resynchronization therapy (CRT), is for people with heart failure due to abnormal work of electrical systems in the heart. The CRT system consists of two components—the pulse generator, or device, and thin, insulated wires called leads. A CRT device delivers tiny amounts of electrical energy to the heart through these leads to restore the normal timing of heartbeats, causing both the ventricles to pump more efficiently. There are two types of CRT devices. One is a special kind of pacemaker called as a cardiac resynchronization therapy pacemaker (CRT-P) or "biventricular pacemaker" [17]. The other is one includes additionally a built-in implantable cardioverter defibrillator (ICD). This device is called a cardiac resynchronization therapy defibrillator (CRT-D), which is used to treat ventricular tachycardia and ventricular fibrillation and avoid sudden cardiac arrest.

The CRT-P device functions like a normal pacemaker to treat slow heart rhythms, as well as delivers small electrical impulses indirectly, however, to the left ventricle to help the both the ventricles contract at the same time.

The CRT-D device combines a dual-chamber pacemaker and a defibrillator. It has the same three leads as a CRT-P, but it can also deliver a high-energy shock to treat fast ventricular arrhythmias (VAs) such as ventricular tachycardia or ventricular fibrillation, which can cause sudden cardiac arrest.

2.5.4 Alternative pacing sites (septum pacing)

It expected that the right ventricular septal pacing is a valid alternative to apical pacing, which most mimics normal physiology. Whether the pacing of right ventricular outflow tract septum (RVOTS) is superior to right ventricular apex (RVA) pacing with respect to cardiac function is still not fully clear. Placing the pacing electrode on the mid-septum may be more challenging than the RVOTS case. Anyway, the septal pacing is of great interest [18]. There is no need to pass the tricuspid valve, but the outcome is similar to right ventricle pacing.

His bundle pacing in humans was first reported in 2000 [19]. Permanent His bundle pacing is an emerging technique to deliver a more physiological pattern of ventricular pacing and has the potential to mitigate the adverse consequences of chronic right ventricular pacing and promote atrioventricular and intraventricular synchrony. His bundle pacing is a technique that uses the native His-Purkinje system to maintain a physiological pattern of ventricular activation. It is a good alternative to RV and biventricular pacing. However, it is currently undergoing clinical trials to verify whether it has any clinical advantages over RVP or biventricular pacing.

3. Radiofrequency ablation to avoid arrhythmias

3.1 The role of ablation in suppressing arrhythmias

Though the electrical pacing enables the suppressing of suddenly appearing arrhythmic phenomena, the most effective outcome can be achieved by using ablation techniques and, sometimes, both ablation and pacing methods together.

Radiofrequency ablation (RFA) has revolutionized the treatment of both supraventricular and ventricular arrhythmias. However, conventional, X-ray-guided mapping techniques have a limited utility in the ablation of more complex arrhythmias, such as in atrial tachycardia, atrial fibrillation (AF), and ventricular tachycardia (VT). By using 3D technologies and catheters permitting faster acquisitions, in association with high-performance imaging techniques, the development of novel mapping systems has led to the overcoming of these limitations [4].

3.2 Atrial fibrillation

In terms of atrial fibrillation, the development of pulmonary vein (PV) electrical isolation has contributed to a significant reduction in the recurrence of AF, particularly in patients with paroxysmal AF. It has previously been shown that the empirical isolation of all four PVs produces better results than the focal ablation of triggers at the PV level or isolation of fewer PVs [4, 5]. Furthermore, in terms of PV isolation, high-power short-duration (HPSD) applications have been shown to be superior to low-power long-duration ablation [20]. In patients with persistent AF and significant remodeling of the left atrium, the use of substrate-based techniques in addition to PV isolation has shown better results [21]. Non-PV electrical activity originating at the level of the Marshall vein, the coronary sinus, and the superior vena cava is another source of AF in some patients; thus, both focal ablation and electrical isolation of these veins have been studied in selected patients [22].

Although previous research has shown an improvement in these patients' ablation results, the long-term impact on outcomes is still unknown, and more research is needed to prove the efficacy of these techniques.

3.3 Ventricular arrhythmias

Ventricular arrhythmias (VAs) can occur on both the normal and abnormal structural hearts. Structural heart diseases are most frequent, and it is well known that cardiomyopathies lead to cardiac injury, which is clinically expressed by VAs. In contrast to ischemic dilated cardiomyopathies (DCMs), the substrate for VAs in nonischemic DCM is not well defined, and patients may present with any type of VAs, including premature ventricular complexes, monomorphic or polymorphic ventricular tachycardia (VT), and ventricular fibrillation [4, 23, 24].

The two main strategies in the ablation of VTs are represented by the detection of the critical isthmus of the VT circuit and the modification of the arrhythmogenic substrate. However, considering the distribution of the scar in patients with DCM, endocardial mapping alone is often insufficient. Previous research demonstrated that combined endocardial and epicardial ablation improved the procedures results, and the mid-term outcomes in patients with previously failed endocardial only ablation and also as a first-line strategy [25, 26].

3.4 Epicardial ablation and high-power short-duration ablations

Two new techniques used for the catheter ablation of cardiac arrhythmias are epicardial ablation and high-power short-duration ablation. The approach in epicardial ablations is similar to that in endocardial ablations, including activation mapping, entrainment mapping, pace mapping, and substrate mapping. However, the optimal access technique and the better prevention of complications remain a subject of future research.

Electrophysiologists should be well-versed in the indications and contraindications of the epicardial approach, as well as different puncture techniques and periprocedural complications. From the posterior approach, anterior approach, needle-in-needle approach, fluoroscopic method, and wire-guided puncture technique, interventionists can select the most appropriate strategy. The surgical method should be considered in the event of pericardial adhesions. Contrast-enhanced computed tomography may have additional benefits, primarily in terms of detecting abnormal anatomical, dynamic, and perfusion characteristics, but also in terms of distinguishing between epicardial fat and scar tissue.

High-power short-duration RFA is defined in a variety of ways, with power ranging from 40 to 90 W and lasting less than 15 seconds per lesion. PV isolation has been a standard strategy for the catheter ablation of AF since the pioneering work of Hassaguerre et al. in 1994 [27]. However, the long procedure times and high rates of PV reconnection that result have sparked interest in using high-power short-duration ablation. To determine the efficacy and safety profile of this novel technique, researchers looked at the particular biophysical ablation characteristics of HPSD ablation.

3.5 Conclusions on radiofrequency ablation

In conclusion, while RFA has demonstrated significant benefits in the treatment of arrhythmias, some issues remain debatable and long-term results are still needed.

4. Summary

Heart rate management and control continues to be a serious problem in medicine, requiring a variety of measures, including the development of implantable cardiac devices and, in particular, the methods and medical indications for their use in the interests of an ever-widening cohort of patients in their various life and health conditions.

Such situations as pacing after syncope, pacing following transcatheter aortic valve implantation, and cardiac resynchronization therapy for both heart failure and the prevention of pacing-induced cardiomyopathy have been of ongoing interest. Automatic pacing rate control responding to the metabolic demand of the organism and pacing in various diseases of the heart, including new diagnostic tools for semiautomatic decision-making on pacing, as well as pacing the His bundle and the left bundle branch, are of intensive recent research.

New techniques are introduced for the catheter ablation of cardiac arrhythmias: epicardial ablation and high-power short-duration radiofrequency ablation. Although both the methods have demonstrated significant benefits in the treatment of arrhythmias, some issues remain debatable and long-term results are still needed. The same goes for the application of both the methods of ablation and pacing, together, although it has been used in medical practice. The combined application of both the methods of ablation and pacing has been used in medical practice, and the effectiveness of the results requires continued research. The optimal access technique and the better prevention of complications remain a subject of future research [28–32].

Finally, the experienced authors of the chapters in the present book will certainly make a significant contribution to the progress of cardiac rhythm management. Moreover, IntechOpen has made substantial contributions to the publishing of scientific and practical results in the field, and a number of books have been issued during the last decade [33–36].

Author details

Mart Min[1]* and Gabriel Cismaru[2]

1 Thomas Johann Seebeck Department of Electronics, Tallinn University of Technology, Tallinn, Estonia

2 5th Department of Internal Medicine, Cardiology-Rehabilitation, Iuliu Hatieganu University of Medicine and Pharmacy, Cluj-Napoca, Romania

*Address all correspondence to: mart.min@taltech.ee

References

[1] Glikson M, Nielsen JC, Kronborg MB, et al. ESC guidelines on cardiac pacing and cardiac resynchronization therapy. European Heart Journal. 2021;**42**(35): 3427-3520. DOI: 10.1093/eurheartj/ehab364

[2] Ellenbogen KA, Wilkoff BL, Kay GN, Lau CP, Auricchio A. Clinical Cardiac Pacing, Defibrillation and Resynchronization Therapy. 5th ed. Philadelphia, PA: Elsevier; 2016. p. 1248

[3] Burri H, Starck C, Auricchio A, et al. EHRA expert consensus statement and practical guide on optimal implantation technique for conventional pacemakers and implantable cardioverter-defibrillators. Europace. 2021;**23**(7):983-1008. DOI: 10.1093/europace/euaa367

[4] Issa ZF, Miller J, Zipe DP. Clinical Arhythmology and Electrophysiology: A Companion to Braunwald's Heart Disease. 3rd ed. Elsevier; 2019. p. 1304

[5] Lau DH, Linz D, Sanders P. New findings in atrial fibrillation mechanisms. Cardiac Electrophysiology Clinics. 2019;**11**(4):563-571. DOI: 10.1016/j.ccep.2019.08.007

[6] Kirk J, Parsonnet V. Cardiac pacing, 1960-1985: A quarter century of medical and industrial innovation. Circulation. 1998;**97**:1978-1991. DOI: 10.1161/01.CIR.97.19.1978

[7] Dell'Orto S, Valli P, Greco EM. Sensors for rate responsive pacing. Indian Pacing and Electrophysiology Journal. 2004;**4**(3):137-145

[8] Trohman G, Huang HD, Larsen T, Krishnan K, Sharma PS. Sensors for rate-adaptive pacing: How they work, strengths, and limitations. Journal of Cardiovascular Electrophysiology. 2020;**31**:3009-3027. DOI: 10.1111/jce.14733

[9] Min M, Parve T, Kink A. Thoracic bioimpedance as a basis for pacing control. Annals of the New York Academy of Sciences. 1999;**873**(1): 155-166. DOI: 10.1111/j.1749-6632.1999.tb09463.x

[10] Shin JW, Yoon JH, Yoon Y. Rate-adaptive pacemaker controlled by motion and respiratory rate using neuro-fuzzy algorithm. Medical & Biological Engineering & Computing. 2001;**39**:694-699. DOI: 10.1007/BF02345444

[11] Hamed B, Abu Ras AK. Fuzzy controller for dual sensors cardiac pacemaker system in pwith Bradycardias at rest. Intelligent Control and Automation. 2015;**6**:159-167. DOI: 10.4236/ica.2015.63016

[12] Min M, Kink A, Parve T, Rätsep I. Bioimpedance based control of rate limits in artificial cardiac pacing. In: Proc. of the IASTED International Conference on Biomedical Engineering (BioMED 2005); 16-18 February 2005; Austria. 2006. pp. 697-703

[13] Tränkler HR, Kanoun O, Min M, Rist M. Smart sensor systems using impedance spectroscopy. Proceedings of the Estonian Academy of Science and Engineering. 2007;**3**(4):455-478

[14] Werner J, Meine M, Hoeland K, Hexamer M, Kloppe A. Sensor and control technology for cardiac pacing. Transactions of the Institute of Measurement and Control Ruhr-University. 2000;**22**(4):289-302

[15] Middour TG, Chen JH, El-Chami MF. Leadless pacemakers: A review of current data and future directions. Progress in Cardiovascular Diseases. 2021;**66**:61-69

[16] Kotalczyk A, Kalarus Z, Wright DJ, Boriani G, Lip G. Cardiac electronic devices: future directions and

challenges. Medical Devices. 2020;**13**:325-338. DOI: 10.2147/MDER.S245625

[17] Medical Advisory Secretariat. Biventricular pacing (cardiac resynchronization therapy): An evidence-based analysis. Ontario Health Technology Assessment Series. 2005;**5**(13):1-60

[18] Worsnick SA, Sharma PS, Vijayaraman P. Right ventricular septal pacing: A Paradigm Shift. The Journal of Innovations in Cardiac Rhythm Management. 2018;**9**(5):3137-3146. DOI: 10.19102/icrm.2018.090501

[19] Hanley A, Singh JP. His bundle pacing: Are we there yet? JACC Clinical Electrophysiology. 2022;**8**(1):70-72. DOI: 10.1016/j.jacep.2021.08.014

[20] Chen CF, Wu J, Jin CL, Liu MJ, Xu YZ. Comparison of high-power short-duration and low-power long-duration radiofrequency ablation for treating atrial fibrillation: Systematic review and meta-analysis. Clinical Cardiology. 2020;**43**(12):1631-1640

[21] Margulescu AD, Mont L. Persistent atrial fibrillation vs paroxysmal atrial fibrillation: differences in management. Expert Review of Cardiovascular Therapy. 2017;**15**(8):601-618. DOI: 10.1080/14779072.2017.1355237

[22] Santangeli P, Marchlinski FE. Techniques for the provocation, localization, and ablation of non-pulmonary vein triggers for atrial fibrillation. Heart Rhythm. 2017;**14**(7):1087-1096. DOI: 10.1016/j.hrthm.2017.02.030

[23] Mathew S, Müller P, Hardy C, Scanavacca MI, Deneke T. Update Ablation ventrikulärer Tachyarrhythmien [Update on ablation of ventricular tachyarrhythmias]. Herzschrittmachertherapie & Elektrophysiologie. 2022;**33**(1):42-48

[24] Kotake Y, Nalliah CJ, Campbell T, Bennett RG, Turnbull S, Kumar S. Comparison of the arrhythmogenic substrate for ventricular tachycardia in patients with ischemic vs non-ischemic cardiomyopathy: Insights from high-density, multi-electrode catheter mapping. Journal of Interventional Cardiac Electrophysiology. 2021

[25] Hanaki Y, Komatsu Y, Nogami A, et al. Combined endo- and epicardial pace-mapping to localize ventricular tachycardia isthmus in ischaemic and non-ischaemic cardiomyopathy. Europace;**202**:euab245

[26] Liuba I, Muser D, Chahal A, et al. Substrate characterization and outcome of catheter ablation of ventricular tachycardia in patients with nonischemic cardiomyopathy and isolated epicardial scar. Circulation. Arrhythmia and Electrophysiology. 2021;**14**(12):e010279. DOI: 10.1161/CIRCEP.121.010279

[27] Hassaguerre M, Marcus F, Poquet F, et al. Electrocardiographic characteristics and catheter ablation of parahissian accessory pathways. Circulation. 1994;**90**:1124-1128. DOI: 10.1161/01.CIR.90.3.1124

[28] Wilner B, Rickard J. Remote monitoring of permanent pacemakers and implantable cardioverter defibrillators. Cardiac Electrophysiology Clinics. 2021;**13**(3):449-457

[29] Taieb DJ, Amara DW. Télésurveillance des stimulateurs et défibrillateurs cardiaques: état des lieux en France et perspectives après le programme ETAPES [Home monitoring follow-up of implantable cardiac defibrillators and stimulators: Current situation in France and possible future after ETAPESprogram]. Annales de Cardiologie et d'Angeiolie (Paris). 2021;**70**(5):322-325

[30] Vij A, Malhotra S. Identifying CRT responders: Moving from electrical to

mechanical dyssynchrony (editorial). Journal of Nuclear Cardiology. 09 February 2022. 3pp. DOI: 10.1007/s12350-022-02914-9

[31] Pavia S, Wilkoff B. The management of surgical complications of pacemaker and implantable cardioverter-defibrillators. Current Opinion in Cardiology. 2001;**16**(1):66-71

[32] Magnusson P, Liv P. Living with a pacemaker: patient-reported outcome of a pacemaker system. BMC Cardiovascular Disorders. 2018;**18**(1):1-7. DOI: 10.1186/s12872-018-0849-6

[33] Das MK. Modern Pacemakers - Present and Future. London, UK: IntechOpen; 2011

[34] Roka A. Current Issues and Recent Advances in Pacemaker Therapy. London, UK: IntechOpen; 2012

[35] Min M. Cardiac Pacemakers - Biological Aspects, Clinical Applications and Possible Complications. London, UK: IntechOpen; 2011

[36] Min M, editor. Cardiac Pacing and Monitoring: New Methods, Modern Devices. London, UK: IntechOpen; 2019

Chapter 2

Pacemakers and Defibrillators Implantation

Kamran Ghods, Mohammad Forozeshfard, Shahrzad Aghaamoo, Narges Amini and Hoda Zangian

Abstract

Since the introduction of pacemakers and defibrillators in the 1960s, many lives have been saved. The technologies used in the development and implantation of such devices are constantly improving, making the procedures increasingly effective and safe. However, the complexity of such implantations makes it one of the most important procedures that need high levels of expertise, knowledge, and experience on the part of the entire surgery team. There is a wide range of devices used for different purposes with various features and characteristics to suit different patients. They range from single-chamber and dual-chamber pacemakers to pulse generators and biventricular pacemakers. The present review chapter seeks to elaborate on the steps of pacemakers and defibrillators implantation, starting from patient selection to post-surgery care and patient education. It outlines all necessary measures in the preoperative, intraoperative, and postoperative stages to ensure the utmost safety, prevent infection, and avoid and treat further complications. The procedures used by our team have demonstrated satisfactory results for patients with a wide variety of conditions.

Keywords: pacemaker, defibrillator, PPM implantation, ICD implantation, anesthesia care

1. Introduction

Cardiac pacemakers (PPM) and implantable cardioverter defibrillators (ICD) are electrophysiological devices that affect different aspects of patients' lives. Research and implantation of PPM and ICD began in the early 1960s. Nowadays, their role in the medical world is widely accepted because of advancements in new technologies and their widespread use, in addition to the improved life expectancy and quality of life in cardiac patients. Few companies produce and supply PPMs and ICDs.

They are a common treatment for irreversible bradycardia and tachyarrhythmias with specific indications. Cardiac pacemakers are made of a pulse generator that produces the electrical current required for the stimulation of the myocardium. One or two electrodes (leads) transmit the electrical activity from the pulse generator to the atrium and ventricle muscle.

As with other surgical procedures, patients require a precise evaluation and special care in preoperative, intraoperative, and postoperative periods. Implantation must be performed under anesthesia care. Anesthesia management plays a vital role as it involves general and local anesthesia.

Undoubtedly, despite the numerous benefits of using PPMs and ICDs, various local and cardiovascular complications may occur. Local complications include pain, swelling, wound hematoma, wound infection, and ipsilateral hemopneumothorax. Cardiovascular complications include lead displacement, lack of sensation and pacing, atrial and ventricular perforation, myocardial hematoma, diaphragmatic pacing, and cardiac tamponade.

Postoperative care should be short-term and long-term, which include wound care, patient education, taking medications, and periodic follow-up. The improvements in the patients' quality of life are very impressive after implantation and could be affected by programming compatibility and psychological, social, and economic behaviors.

2. Patient selection

Patients are nominated for pacemaker (PPM) and implantable cardiac defibrillator (ICD) implantation according to the patient's history, symptoms and signs, physical examinations and other documents, cardiac imaging (echocardiography) in case of bradycardia/tachycardia, and based on the 2021 European Society of Cardiology (ESC) guidelines on cardiac pacing and cardiac resynchronization therapy, which was developed by the Task Force on cardiac pacing and cardiac resynchronization therapy [1].

A majority of all pacemaker implantations are indicated to patients above 60 years old. After admitting the patient and obtaining informed consent, the necessary blood tests, chest X-ray, and electrocardiography are taken, and then the patient is prepared for the procedure. The patient is transferred to the electrophysiology laboratory, where it is essential to have properly functioning equipment. In addition, standard air conditioning is crucial in controlling air infections. In the era of the Covid-19 pandemic, we need to consider health protocols and guidelines for the personal protection of staff and patients. If there is no emergency condition, pacemaker and ICD implantation should be delayed; otherwise, we must follow all the instructions and protocols related to the prevention of the disease.

3. Types of devices

- Single-chamber pacemaker, which has one lead that connects the pulse generator to the right ventricle or atrium.

- Dual-chamber pacemaker, which has two leads that connect the pulse generator to the right atrium and ventricle, modifying the rhythm of the heart.

- Biventricular pacemaker, which is also known as a cardiac resynchronization therapy (CRT) device and has three leads connecting the pulse generator to the right atrium and both ventricles, which is indicated in advanced heart failure.

- Implantable cardioverter defibrillators (ICD), which include single-chamber and dual-chamber.

- Pulse generators, which are implanted subcutaneously and their leads are divided into three categories: endocardial, epicardial, and subcutaneous. We generally apply endocardial leads with extensive experience in this field of medicine.

- A new generation of PPM was introduced by Medtronic Company in 2016, offering leadless transcatheter pacing systems for bradyarrhythmia management. It is applied percutaneously via a minimally invasive approach, directly into the right ventricle, and does not require leads.

4. Surgical instruments and equipment

In the setting of device implantation by a cardiac surgeon, the required instruments for better management of the procedure are as illustrated in **Figure 1**. We have achieved desirable results using standard surgical techniques for gentle and homeostatic manipulation of tissue.

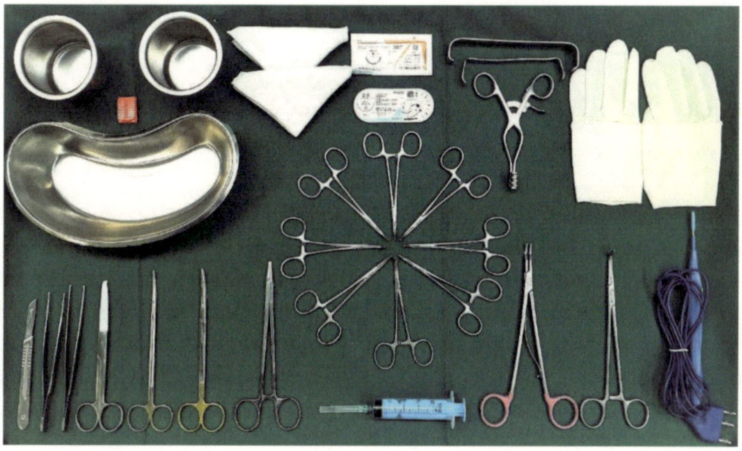

Figure 1.
Surgical instruments required for surgical pacemaker and ICD implantation.

5. Anesthesia considerations in patients undergoing PPM and ICD implantation

5.1 Pre-anesthesia care

The electrophysiology laboratory (EP lab) should be equipped with the following: anesthesia machine, air mask bag unit (patient-ventilator), electrocardiogram (ECG or EKG), pulse oximetry, defibrillators, emergency trolley, suction machine, external pacing equipment, capnography, airway management equipment. Moreover, emergency medications, including dantrolene for malignant hyperthermia, intralipid for toxicity due to local anesthetics, and antidotes drugs (naloxone, neostigmine, sugammadex, flumazenil), resuscitation drugs (epinephrine, atropine), anesthetics (propofol, etomidate), sedatives (midazolam), analgesics (fentanyl), antiarrhythmic drugs, and inotropes should be available. In addition to inspecting and preparing the equipment, an experienced and trained staff (including an anesthetic team who are sufficiently skilled in resuscitation) should be present. All patients seeking pacemaker and ICD implantation require preoperative evaluations, including (ECG), chest radiograph, blood tests (complete blood count and differentiation, BUN, CR, PT, PTT, INR), and electrolyte levels (K, Na, Ca) (**Figure 2**).

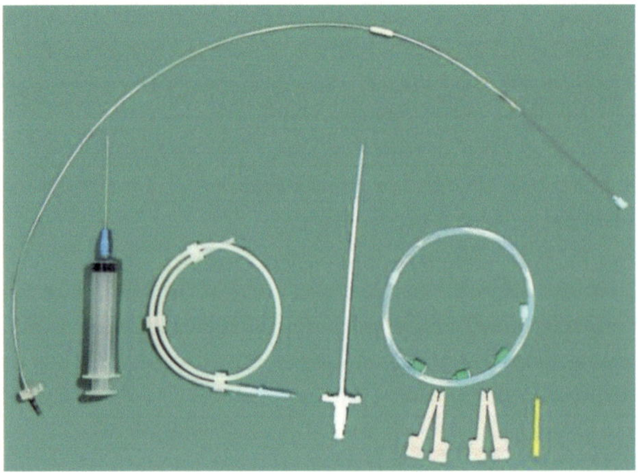

Figure 2.
Instrument setup for lead implantation based on Seldinger technique.

5.2 Preoperative evaluation

1. Medical history and medications: The patient's past medical history (type of arrhythmia, history of myocardial infarction (MI), stroke, heart failure, valvular heart disease, previous cardiac revascularization, obstructive sleep apnea (OSA), COPD (chronic obstructive pulmonary disease), difficult intubation), ECG, current medications (anticoagulants, antithrombotic drugs, antihypertensive drugs, antiarrhythmic agents, diuretics), and any medication associated with the prolongation of VT (ventricular tachycardia) should be carefully evaluated.

2. Physical examination: The patient must be examined for devices such as IABP (intra-aortic balloon pump), VAD (ventricular assist device), other implantable heart devices; surgical scar; symptoms of compensated heart failure, vital signs, electrolytes, kidney function, and TTE (transthoracic echocardiogram) to rule out heart thrombosis and assess ventricular function and valvular heart disease.

3. The procedure should be explained to the patient to reduce her/his anxiety before getting informed consent.

4. The American Board of Anesthesiology recommends that patients should not eat solid food for at least 8 hours before a procedure and should not drink even clear liquids for at least 2 hours prior.

5.3 Anesthesia care

The anesthesia team's performance is vital for the management of patients with multiple risk factors and older ages. The medical team must be prepared for potentially catastrophic events such as cardiac arrest, cardiac tamponade, and unstable arrhythmias. Therefore, make sure that surgical instruments and anesthesia support measures are ready for emergency sternotomy.

In these patients, the relationship between the EP physician and the anesthesiologist is crucial. The type of anesthesia is determined based on the patient's medical history and condition and might involve monitored anesthesia care (MAC), sedation, regional anesthesia, or general anesthesia. The patient's position is usually supine so that the right or left shoulder (according to the surgeon's decision) is elevated by a pad. Also, the positions of the head and neck are very important and should be in a way that the patient feels comfortable. The patient's head is rotated to the opposite side of the surgical site for easier access to the subclavian vein. The airway should be easily accessible because of intravenous sedation. Most patients undergo local anesthesia with intravenous sedation by applying oxygen through a non-rebreather mask. The hands should be neutrally placed on either side. Standard vital signs monitoring is performed with ECG, pulse oximetry, non-invasive blood pressure monitoring (NIBP), and capnography.

The patient should be constantly monitored for airway obstruction and respiratory failure regardless of the anesthetic technique. In case of airway obstruction, the chin-lift and jaw-thrust maneuvers are immediately performed. Excessive restlessness, anxiety, and pain intolerance due to electric shock are the reasons for choosing general anesthesia with intravenous sedation. The arterial line should be established for patients with severe conditions.

5.4 Post-anesthesia care

Postoperative care and monitoring are mandatory due to the probability of surgical and anesthesia complications caused by an underlying disease.

6. Implantation procedure

6.1 Antibiotic prophylaxis

According to the European Society of Cardiology (ESC) guidelines on cardiac pacing and cardiac resynchronization therapy, antibiotic prophylaxis is recommended in PPM and ICD implantation procedures to prevent *Staphylococcus aureus* species. The risk of infection is significantly reduced with a single dose of prophylactic antibiotic (cefazolin 1–2 g I.V. or flucloxacillin 1–2 g I.V.) applied within 30–60 minutes before the procedure [2].

6.2 Surgical incision

To get better anatomical access to the central vessels of the heart, we use local anesthesia with the administration of 4.5 mg/kg of 2% lidocaine for the sake of the patient's comfort. Then, an incision is made (2.5 inches for PPM and 3.5–4 inches for ICD) with a number 15 blade in the distal third of the right infraclavicular region of the anterior chest wall (**Figure 3**). The subcutaneous tissue is opened and dissected in a layer under the pectoralis major fascia with accurate homeostasis using electrocautery (**Figure 4**). The development of a subpectoral pocket may be advisable in patients with a low body-mass index and for esthetic reasons.

6.3 Central venous access

Tran's venous lead implantation is commonly performed through venous access via the right or left cephalic, subclavian or axillary vein. In case clinical signs of a venous occlusion of deep veins of the upper extremity are observed, preoperative assessment (colored Doppler sonogram, venography, or chest CT scan) may be useful to determine optimal venous access or find an alternative access way.

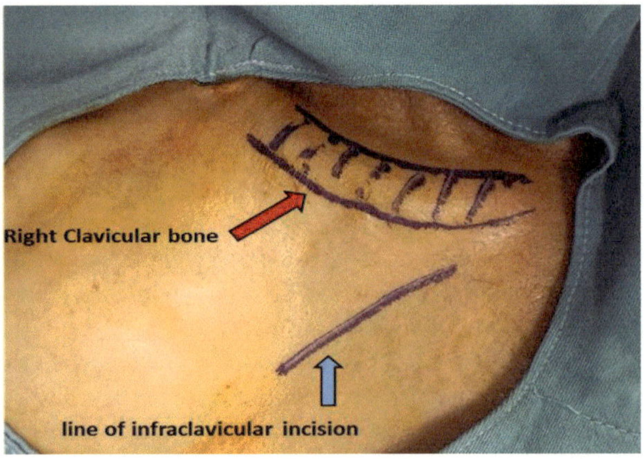

Figure 3.
Right infraclavicular incision region and marker.

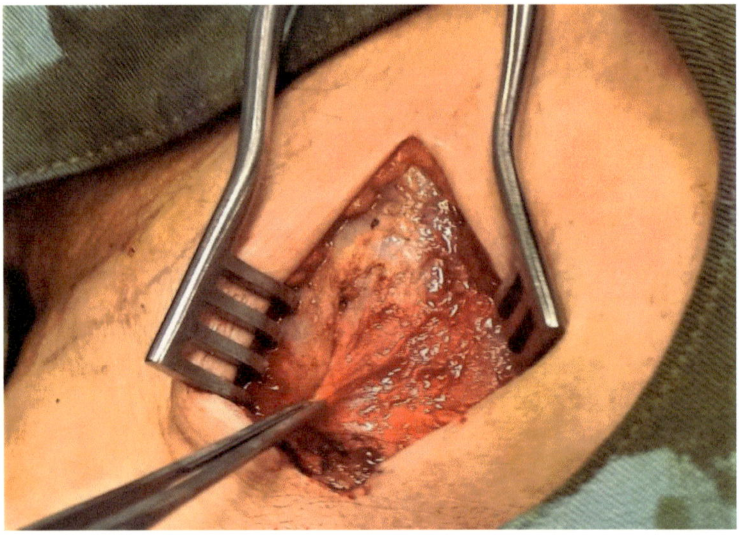

Figure 4.
Right pectoralis major fascia.

By applying the Seldinger technique, we first enter the right subclavian vein using a needle and syringe. Then, we insert a guide wire through the subclavian vein, superior vena cava, and the right atrium, determining the proper location using fluoroscopy. The lead introducer (7 French or 9 French) is sent through a guide wire and then the right ventricular (RV) lead (58 cm length) is passed through the introducer to the RV apex or interventricular septum, latter for patients who need more RV and LV contractile synchronization (**Figure 5**). The second guide wire is passed through the subclavian vein to the right atrium, and the 52 cm length lead is placed inside the right atrial appendage in the same manner and analyzed by a pacemaker programmer. An alternative technique is cephalic vein cut-down, which is occasionally performed by surgeons to reduce side effects. Subclavian vein access is associated with a 7.8-fold increased risk of pneumothorax [1]. In case subclavian venous access is not feasible, transfemoral lead implantation is alternatively performed, or leadless PPM or epicardial lead should be considered.

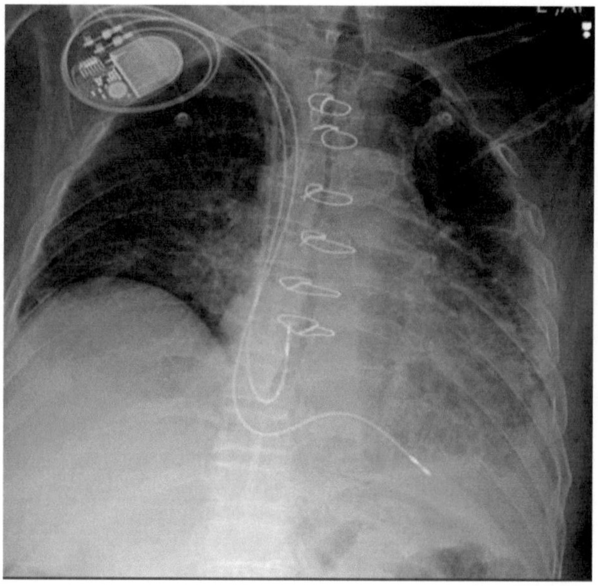

Figure 5.
Proper position of activated leads in right atrial appendage and right ventricular apex with noticeable tip position.

7. Analysis

7.1 Initial analysis

Pre-activation lead analyses have revealed the proper lead location and features as follows:

- Right ventricular (R) wave sensing: 5–20 Millivolts
- Right atrial (P) wave sensing: 1–5 Millivolts
- Lead impedance (resistance): 200–2000 Ohms
- Pacing threshold: <1 Millivolts

After initial analysis and making sure about proper leads position, the ventricular and atrial leads are screwed (activated), fixed, and re-analyzed. The same steps are carried out for RV lead-coiled (58 or 65 cm length) and should be more cautious of which can cause more endocardial trauma to the heart structures because of more stiffness. The ST-segment elevation (STE) diagram is checked in pace maker programmer. After screwing, the suture sleeve of the lead should be tied with a 3-0 black silk suture to pectoralis major fascia. Thus, each lead is fixed in two areas, the endocardium (screwed) and on the pectoralis major muscle. In the next step, after changing the surgical gloves and irrigating the subcutaneous pocket with a normal saline solution ensuring strict observance of sterility, the outer end of the RV and RA leads is connected to the pulse generator and securely screwed. The pulse generator is then placed in the subcutaneous pocket, so that the outer end of the leads is rounded beneath the generator with no bending and kinking. The PPM and the ICD function should be programmed using a sterile head or wireless programmer. The wound is repaired in three layers following irrigation and homeostasis. The patient is then transferred to the recovery room for further vital signs monitoring. A sandbag weighing 1–3 kg can be placed on the wound site to prevent hematoma, and finally admitted to the OHICU. On the same day, chest X-ray and ECG tests are performed. Prior to discharge, we should make sure about wound healing and proper functioning of device (final analysis) and patient's general conditions to be satisfactory and provide the patient with all required information about new lifestyle and device dependency, accordingly those patients with ICD should be trained and aware of the painfulness of related shock. Scheduling for further visits and analyses is recommended.

7.2 Final analysis

Final analyses consist of the following items to achieve optimum results:

- Mood determination as recommended by the North American Society of Pacing and Electrophysiology/British Pacing and Electrophysiology Group (NASPE/BPEG)
- Lower rate limit
- Pacing amplitude
- Pulse width
- Sensitivity
- Upper rate limit for atrial track
- For ICD: determination of the VT and VF zone
- Configuration of leads (bipolar and unipolar)

8. Complications

Implantation can be associated with as many complications as other cardiovascular surgeries in the preoperative phase. In addition, the presence of the device inside the vessel and the heart itself is associated with early and late complications. The majority of complications occur in the hospital or within a few months after the surgery. Therefore, the cardiac surgeon should be trained about the proper management of complications and treating life-threatening conditions, and obviously, the more experienced the surgeon, the fewer the complications. The complexity of the device generally increases the potential risks. Nowadays, the device pocket is considered a source of major complications. Therefore, preventing pocket hematoma and infection has become a standard care measure. Complications are now described as early and late.

8.1 Early complications

Early complications include the following:

- Pain (surgical site or device-related)
- Wound bleeding: 0.5–3% [3]

- Pocket hematoma: accounting for over 3% of complications [4]
- Pericardial effusion or tamponade
- Pneumothorax: 0.5–2.2%
- Coronary sinus dissection or perforation: 0.7–2.1%
- Hemothorax: 0.1%
- Subclavian artery puncture
- Lead perforation: 0.8% [5]

8.2 Late complications

Late complications include the following:

- Superficial infection: 1.2%
- Pocket infection: 1.3% [4]
- Diaphragmatic pacing requiring reintervention: 0.55%
- Deep venous thrombosis
- Upper extremity edema
- Endocarditis
- Programming failure (vertigo, headache, palpitation, and blurred vision)
- Wound dehiscence
- Lead fracture
- Inappropriate shocks
- Skin erosion
- Pericarditis
- Lead dislodgment (**Figure 6**)
- Mortality (<30 days): 0.8–1.4%
- Systemic infection: 0.5–1.2%
- Tricuspid regurgitation: 16% [6]
- Pacemaker syndrome: 5–80% [7]
- Psychological problems: up to 35% of people develop anxiety disorder following ICD placement, although disabling problems necessitating admission are fairly uncommon [8]

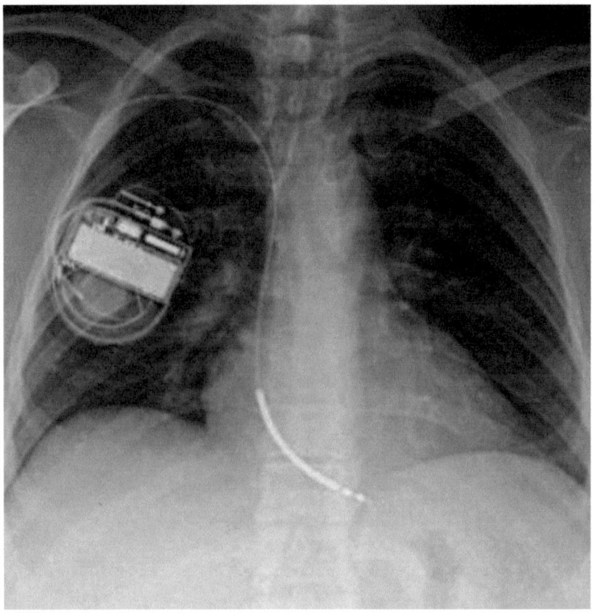

Figure 6.
Right ventricular lead-coiled dislodgment as late complication.

- Economic problems
- Replacement of pulse generator (4%) and with one or more additional lead insertions: 15.3% [1]
- Phlebitis or thrombophlebitis: 30–50% [9]

9. Post-discharge care and education points

The following points should be reminded and taught to patients for the post-discharge period.

- Keep the wound clean and dry. If you notice a swollen wound, seek medical help.
- You can take a shower 48 hours after the operation.
- Do not move your pacemaker under the skin and manipulate it.
- Do not move the arm on the same side of pacemaker implantation for up to 24 hours.
- You should not lift the arm above the shoulder for up to 4 weeks.
- The patient is instructed to seek medical support in case of fever and any discharge from the wound.
- Consume the medications according to the physician's instructions.
- The patient should not lift more than 4–7 kg.

- Avoid hitting, pressing, and sleeping on the operated site.
- Before going to spaces with strong magnetic fields and electrical circuits, consult with the treating physician and be analyzed if necessary.
- For periodic analyses, plan for 1 week, 1 month, 3 months, and 6 months later.
- Always carry your pacemaker profile card with you.

10. Conclusion

This review chapter provided a detailed outline of all the required steps involved in the implantation of pacemakers and defibrillators. The sensitive nature of the procedure requires an in-depth and careful analysis of the patient's medical history and present conditions to minimize the risk of future complications.

Extensive care and caution should be practiced in preoperative, intra-operative, and postoperative courses to ensure the risk of early complications, especially infection, are reduced. Patients need detailed instructions to learn how to live with their implanted devices. Patient-physician interaction would earn suitable long-life results.

Conflict of interest

None declared.

Author details

Kamran Ghods[1*], Mohammad Forozeshfard[2], Shahrzad Aghaamoo[3], Narges Amini[4] and Hoda Zangian[4]

1 Clinical Research Development Unit, Kowsar Hospital, Semnan University of Medical Sciences, Semnan, Iran

2 Cancer Research Center, Semnan University of Medical Sciences, Semnan, Iran

3 Abnormal Uterine Bleeding Research Center, Semnan University of Medical Sciences, Semnan, Iran

4 Department of Cardiac Surgery, Kowsar Hospital, Semnan University of Medical Sciences, Semnan, Iran

*Address all correspondence to: kamran1230@yahoo.com

References

[1] Glikson M, Nielsen JC, Kronborg MB, Michowitz Y, Auricchio A, Barbash IM, et al. 2021 ESC guidelines on cardiac pacing and cardiac resynchronization therapy. European Heart Journal. 2021;**42**(35):3427-3520. DOI: 10.1093/eurheartj/ehab364

[2] De Oliveira JC, Martinelli M, Nishioka SA, Varejao T, Uipe D, Pedrosa AA, et al. Efficacy of antibiotic prophylaxis before the implantation of pacemakers and cardioverter-defibrillators: Results of a large, prospective, randomized, double-blinded, placebo-controlled trial. Circulation. Arrhythmia and Electrophysiology. 2009;**2**:29-34

[3] Nichols C, Vose J. Incidence of bleeding-related complications during primary implantation and replacement of cardiac implantable electronic devices. Journal of the American Heart Association. 2017;**6**(1):e004263

[4] Mulpuru SK, Madhavan M, McLeod CJ, Cha YM, Friedman PA. Cardiacpacemakers: Function, troubleshooting, and management: Part 1 of a 2-part series. Journal of the American College of Cardiology. 2017;**69**(2):189-210

[5] Chao JA, Firstenberg MS. Delayed pacemaker lead perforations: Why unusual presentations should prompt an early multidisciplinary team approach. International Journal of Critical Illness and Injury Science. 2017;7(1):65-68

[6] Delling F, Hassan Z, Piatkowski G, et al. Tricuspid regurgitation and mortality in patients with transvenous permanent pacemaker leads. The American Journal of Cardiology. 2016;**117**(6):988-992. DOI: 10.1016/j.amjcard.2015.12.038

[7] Ausubel K, Furman S. The pacemaker syndrome. Annals of Internal Medicine. 1985;**103**(3):420-429. DOI: 10.7326/0003-4819-103-3-420

[8] Kamphuis HC, de Leeuw JR, Derksen R, Hauer RN, Winnubst JA. Implantable cardioverter defibrillator recipients: Quality of life in recipients with and without ICD shock delivery: A prospective study. Europace. 2003;**5**(4):381-389

[9] Marx J, Walls R, Hockberger E. Rosen's Emergency Medicine: Concepts and Clinical Practice E-Book. 9th ed. Elsevier Health Sciences; March 9, 2017; eBook ISBN:9780323390163

Chapter 3

Operation of Implantable Cardiac Devices in Hyperbaric Conditions

Jacek Kot

Abstract

Implantable devices, including Implantable Cardiac Defibrillators (ICD) and Pacemakers (PM), are being seen with increasing frequency in patients wanting to conduct recreational diving or referred for Hyperbaric Oxygen Therapy (HBOT). Under hyperbaric conditions, these devices are at risk of malfunction, mostly by changes of ambient pressure. In some cases, manufacturers publish information on how their devices operate under increased pressure. Unfortunately, this is not always the case, and for other devices, someone must perform an individual risk-benefit analysis specific for single patient and his/her implanted device. In case of medical treatment, such analysis must take into account the patient's clinical condition, the indication for HBOT, and the capability of the HBOT facility for monitoring and intervention in the chamber.

Keywords: diving, hyperbaric medicine, oxygen, defibrillator

1. Introduction

The hyperbaric chamber is an active medical device, which is potentially hazardous taking into accounts its application and exposure of people inside to increased ambient pressure and increased partial pressure of oxygen. Typically, in most clinical indications, the internal pressure of 2.5 absolute atmosphere (ATA) (equivalent to 15 m of sea water [msw]) is used, with the range from 1.5 to 6.0 ATA (equivalent to 5–50 msw), for a period of 60 min, with the range from 30 to 120 min, as depending on the specific hyperbaric center [1]. Regardless of using the monoplace chamber, where patient is left alone within the pressure vessel, or in multiplace chamber, where patient is staying in the larger internal space together with medical attendant, as with other patients, if so organized, in all cases, any medical device, either external to the patients or implanted, including Implantable Cardiac Defibrillators (ICD) and Pacemakers (PM), is exposed to increased ambient pressure.

Use of other medical devices for therapeutic purpose in the hyperbaric chamber is also related with additional hazards due to increased pressure, oxygen-enriched atmosphere, electricity, and confined space. Therefore, every medical device introduced into the hyperbaric chamber should be designed in that way that its use in the hyperbaric chamber does not create significant risk of malfunction, damage, or ignition of fire in the hyperbaric environment; this should be certified by the manufacturer for specific conditions (working pressure, maximum allowable content of oxygen, temperature, and humidity). Unfortunately, until now only few medical devices are specifically designed for usage in hyperbaric chambers.

Therefore, medical providers often need to conduct themselves appropriate assessment of the medical equipment needed for continuation of intensive or general care during hyperbaric treatment.

2. Risk management process

In Europe, as well as in the rest of the world, the general risk management process applicable for all medical devices is described in the ISO EN 14971 [2]. This concerns also ICDs and PMs. Detailed recommendations for medical devices used specifically in hyperbaric chamber systems are presented in the Annex B of the European Norm CEN EN14931 [3]. This Annex includes a description of all potential hazards that can be created by the use of specific medical devices, as well as the risks induced by them inside medical hyperbaric chambers. Moreover, in order to ensure the highest possible level of safety of the patient treated with the Hyperbaric Oxygen Therapy (HBOT) and the attendants, recommendations are given to both manufacturers of such devices and medical users of hyperbaric installations [3].

Generally speaking, there are three hazards related to the use of medical devices in the hyperbaric chamber:

1. An increased ambient pressure and changes of pressure during compression and decompression can significantly affect mechanical parts of the item, leading to distortion of its structure or even damaged and/or performance deterioration of the medical devices, which have been designed and manufactured for use at normobaric pressure.

2. An increased fractional amount of oxygen, either locally, as so-called "oxygen clouds," or generally in mixed chamber atmosphere, creates risk for fire, especially if combined with a source of ignition, e.g., local overheating or sparks and combustible products (e.g., oil, grease)—see below.

3. The electricity used for medical devices in the hyperbaric environment creates a risk for fire as a potential source of ignition when sparking or overheating.

The preferred method of using medical devices inside hyperbaric chambers is having manufacturer's clearance for specific ambient conditions, confirmed by the appropriate certificated, e.g., "CE certificate" in European Union. However, there are some cases when the medical devices need to be introduced into the hyperbaric environment, but the manufacturer does not certify them for use in such conditions. In those cases, the user of the device (staff of hyperbaric centers) must conduct the safety evaluation before introducing it to the hyperbaric environment. This process includes at least checking the structure of the device, taking into account:

1. Increased ambient pressure and its changes to make sure that it is pressure-resistant or at least it does not have any sealed compartments, which could be mechanically damaged;

2. Increased oxygen fraction in the ambient atmosphere to ensure that it does not contain any material that is either non-compatible with oxygen or easily combustible;

3. Electrical power supply to ensure that it does not use high energy (both with voltage and current) inside the hyperbaric chamber.

In case of any doubt, the use of this medical device in hyperbaric chamber should be abandoned.

3. The practice

The number of patients with implanted pacemakers (PM) and automatic implanted cardiac defibrillators (AICD) treated inside hyperbaric chambers for other medical reasons is growing.

Internal cardiac pacemaker cans are semi-rigid pieces of equipment, providing to some degree both water tightness to the internal circuits and protection against external pressure. It seems logical that due to different compressibility, use of a resin-filled ICD/PM should be safer than a gas-filled model [4]. According to general opinion, internal cardiac pacemakers are unaffected by the hyperbaric environment [5]. However—obviously—the pressure resistance can be true only for limited range of pressures. During the ISO-compatible ETO-standard sterilization process, the pressure is from 1.7 up to 2.5 ATA (7–15 msw); therefore, all the devices sterilized by this method are unintentionally tested for at least such overpressure [6]. Some implanted devices were used to at least 2.4 ATA (14 msw) [7, 8]. There are also reports that all pacemakers tested by the authors were adequate to treatment pressure below 3 ATA (20 msw), and some even to 7 ATA (60 msw) [9].

One of the ICD/PM manufacturers officially reported that their devices "should operate normally up to 49.5 feet of seawater (2.5 ATA, 15 msw) and will begin to significantly deform at pressures near 132 feet of seawater (5 ATA, 40 msw)" and that "No loss or degradation of output operation was observed in any of the devices tested; however, rate responsive pacing began to diminish at pressures in excess of 66 feet of seawater (3 ATA, 20 msw), which caused the devices to pace at the programmed lower rate. The loss of rate responsive pacing was observed to be temporary; activity pacing returned at lesser pressures" [10].

There was a suspicion that if ICD leads are damaged, ignition could occur if the ICD discharges, so some experts advised that defibrillation mode of the ICDs should be deactivated before HBOT [11].

Indeed, the question whether dangerous electrical arcing harmful for either patient or any medical attendant touching him/her can occur in case of implanted device malfunction during resuscitation in the hyperbaric chamber is a vital one.

In the literature, there are some reported events concerning skin burns due to faulty automatic ICDs at normobaric conditions [12]. There are also some reports of electric shocks passed to the rescuer doing chest compressions while performing cardiopulmonary resuscitation (CPR) out of the hyperbaric chamber [13–15]. In the statement from the one ICD manufacturer, there is a note that "Although we are not aware of any reported incidences of ICD shock triggered ignition, and do not believe this to be of significant risk, it may be advisable to disable defibrillation therapies, pending further study to the contrary, while patients are undergoing hyperbaric treatments" [10].

Based on results of experiments performed on dogs using energy of 30 joules by the internal defibrillator [16] as well as the analysis of the worst-case scenario (Dr. Jake Freiberger, Duke University, USA, personal communication), the energy released from the malfunctioned ICD should not exceed 0.374 W, which is well below NFPA equipment guideline limit of 0.5 W for any medical devices entering the hyperbaric chamber [17]. In summary, the risk of fire caused by the electric arc initiated by the malfunction ICD/PM can be made negligible, even if the defibrillation option is left ON during hyperbaric session. But, in fact, ICD defibrillation during HBOT has not been reported, nor tested.

In the largest study concerning independent testing of commercially available cardiac pacemakers [18], 40 separate pacemakers supplied by four different manufacturers were exposed to liquid pressurization in a small hyperbaric chamber up to 4 ATA (30 msw) and 7 ATA (60 msw). Throughout the testing, no recording of arrhythmia, reprogramming, or any other electronic dysfunction was noted. During the pressurization period, a transient (<90 s duration) increase of the pacing rate of some rate-responsive pacemakers was noted. This pacing rate increase, which was sometimes large (up to +40 beats per minute), slowed down spontaneously. The mechanical results related to the can's deformation showed that all casings were reversibly distorted during pressurizations. No permanent deformation was observed at pressures up to 4 ATA (30 msw). However, after the 7 ATA test (60 msw), 65% of the devices tested were significantly deformed in the electronic part of the device (**Figure 1**), whereas the battery part was not significantly altered. No connector deformation or damage was noted.

The authors concluded that there was good electronic tolerance for all devices both during and after hyperbaric tests. Also, there was a good tolerance of all the devices studied to a liquid environment with a good water tightness up to 7 ATA (60 msw). So, the risk of dysfunction of a device related to penetration of liquids into the can appears to be very low. And this was in accordance with the data published also on other implantable devices [19].

In the literature, one can find also summary list of ICD/PM, which have been used under different pressures showing no obvious malfunction [20], as well as lists of devices from different manufacturers, which were permitted by the manufacturer to be exposed in real HBOT sessions based on individual requests from referring physicians [21]. These cover different pressures from 1 ATA to 7 ATA (from 0 msw to 60 msw) in most cases.

The list of implanted devices, which have been already exposed to some degree for the hyperbaric conditions, will never be exhaustive, as every year some new devices are showing on the market, and some patients with new devices are referred to the hyperbaric facilities. Moreover, the fact that in some patients, implanted devices works fine, does not mean that it concerns all the items from the series.

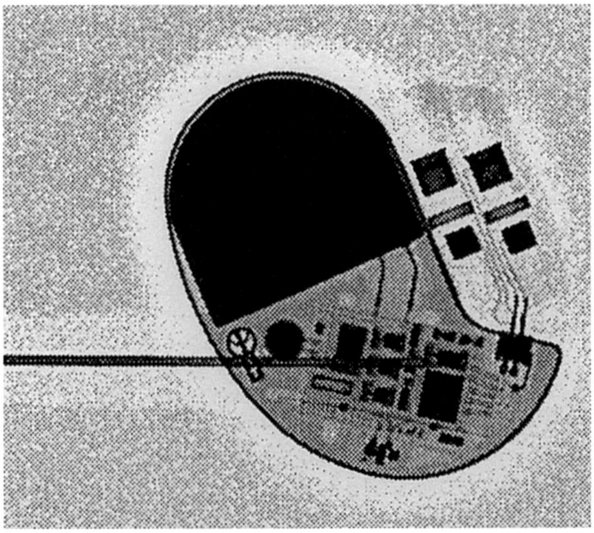

Figure 1.
X-ray picture of a pacemaker. Note maximal deformation, which is located at the tip of the needle (from [18], with copyrights).

There are several options on how to manage those implanted devices, which are not yet officially approved for hyperbaric conditions [22]. First option is to request manufacturer to support the hyperbaric facility staff with the written opinion about the compatibility of the ICD with the specific hyperbaric conditions (absolute pressure, time of exposure, and number of planned hyperbaric sessions). This can be applicable, if the clinical indication is not acute one, but chronic, when the start of HBOT can be safely delayed. For such approach, it is necessary to have direct contact with the ICD manufacturer's representative in the country, as for international use, there is no communication channel available.

The other option, used also in our hyperbaric center, is to perform the risk assessment by the hyperbaric medicine specialist, which will consider the fact that most modern compact ICD are internally pressure resistant, at least due to the sterilization process (see above). So, the residual risk for ICD failure is low and should be accepted by most patients having obvious clinical indications for using HBOT [23]. Such approach seems valid at least until the pressure of 4 ATA (30 msw of depth). In most reports, the extension of the limit to 7 ATA (60 msw) results in mechanical reversible distortion of the device can with functional disturbances, but without any reported permanent failures in most of modern devices.

Nevertheless, it is highly advisable to constantly monitor ECG of patients with implanted pacemakers and cardiac defibrillators during every HBO session [22]. Every hyperbaric facility should have implemented the protocol for clinical management in case of ICD failure during the hyperbaric treatment. This should cover either switching off the internal device not working properly or external pacing if necessary for life threating situations.

4. Conclusions

Implantable devices, including Implantable Cardiac Defibrillators (ICD) and Pacemakers (PM), are being seen with increasing frequency in patients wanting to conduct recreational diving or referred for Hyperbaric Oxygen Therapy (HBOT). Considering the intrinsic properties of the modern implantable devices, it seems that the residual risk for malfunction while being exposed to maximum pressure of 4 ATA, equivalent to the depth of 30 msw, is extremely low. Greater pressures up to 7 ATA (equivalent to the depth of 60 msw) increase the risk of temporarily deterioration with degradation of the performance. Higher pressures, unlikely to be used either in modern HBOT or in recreational conservative diving, can cause permanent damage of the device; unless specifically tested and confirmed by the manufacturer, such exposures should be avoided.

Conflict of interest

I declare no conflict of interest.

Author details

Jacek Kot
National Center for Hyperbaric Medicine, Institute of Maritime and Tropical Medicine, Medical University of Gdansk, Gdynia, Poland

*Address all correspondence to: jacek.kot@gumed.edu.pl

References

[1] Mathieu D. Handbook on Hyperbaric Medicine. Netherlands: Springer; 2006

[2] ISO-EN-14971. Medical Devices—Application of Risk Management to Medical Devices. 2007

[3] CEN-EN-14931. Pressure vessels for human occupancy (PVHO)—Multi-place pressure chamber systems for hyperbaric therapy—Performance, safety requirements and testing. 2006

[4] Kratz JM, Blackburn JG, Leman RB, Crawford FA. Cardiac pacing under hyperbaric conditions. The Annals of Thoracic Surgery. 1983;**36**(1):66-68

[5] Kindwall EP. Contraindications and side effects to hyperbaric oxygen treatment. In: Kindwall EP, editor. Hyperbaric Medicine Practice. Flagstaff, USA: Best Publishing Company; 1999. pp. 83-98

[6] Wonhas C, Wonhas-Thiele H. Safety in hyperbaric oxygen therapy (HBO) also for patients with implanted pacemakers (PM)? Undersea & Hyperbaric Medicine. 1998;**25** (suppl):15

[7] Simmons S, Zmaeff J. Review of implanted cardiac rhythm devices in the hyperbaric chamber. Undersea & Hyperbaric Medicine. 2001;**28**(suppl):101

[8] Simmons C, Zmaeff J. Review of implanted cardiac rhythm devices in the hyperbaric chamber. Undersea & Hyperbaric Medicine. 2001;**28**(suppl): 84-85

[9] Simmons C. Review of permanent pacemakers in hyperbaric chambers. Undersea & Hyperbaric Medicine. 1998;**25**(suppl):14

[10] MEDTRONIC. Medtronic statement, Rev. A. 1. 2010

[11] Schmitz S, Churchill S, Weaver LK. Hyperbaric oxygen in patients with implanted cardiac defibrillators and pacemakers. Undersea & Hyperbaric Medicine. 2006;**33**(5):349

[12] Landaluce CG, Lozano IF, Ramos JE, Urda VC, Pereira EP. A singular skin burn. Pacing and Clinical Electrophysiology. 2010;**33**(10):1288

[13] Wallace CK. In-hospital cardiopulmonary resuscitation. The New England Journal of Medicine. 2009;**361**(17):1708; author reply –9

[14] Clements PA. Hazards of performing chest compressions in collapsed patients with internal cardioverter defibrillators. Emergency Medicine Journal. 2003;**20**(4):379-380

[15] Siniorakis E, Hardavella G, Arvanitakis S, Roulia G, Voutas P, Karidis C. Accidental shock to rescuer from an implantable cardioverter defibrillator. Resuscitation. 2009; **80**(3):293-294

[16] Niwano S, Kojima J, Inuo K, Saito J, Kashiwa T, Suyama M, et al. Measurement of body surface energy leakage of defibrillation shock by an implantable cardioverter defibrillator. Pacing and Clinical Electrophysiology. 2002;**25**(8):1212-1218

[17] NFPA-99. Health Care Facilities Code. NFPA; 2005

[18] Lafay V, Trigano JA, Gardette B, Micoli C, Carre F. Effects of hyperbaric exposures on cardiac pacemakers. British Journal of Sports Medicine. 2008;**42**(3):212-216. discussion 6

[19] Wonhas C, Wonhas-Thiele H, Mueller A. Implanted cardiac defibrillator (ICD) and pacemaker (PM) after longtime hyperbaric oxygentherapy. Biotronik Phylax AV

and Inos Plus. Undersea & Hyperbaric Medicine. 2000;**27**(suppl):32

[20] Kot J. Medical equipment for multiplace hyperbaric chambers. Part 1: Devices for monitoring and cardiac support. European Journal of Underwater and. Hyperbaric Medicine. 2005;**6**:115-120

[21] Novotný Š, editor. Zásady pro léčebnou hyperbaroxii u pacientů s implantovaným kardiostimulátorem a defibrilátorem. Ostravské dny hyperbarické medicíny. Hukvaldy: Česká republika; 2012

[22] Kot J, Houman R, Müller P. Hyperbaric chamber and equipment. In: Mathieu D, editor. Handbook on Hyperbaric Medicine. Dordrecht: Springer; 2006. pp. 611-636

[23] Mathieu D, Ratzenhofer-Komenda B, Kot J. Hyperbaric oxygen therapy for intensive care patients: Position statement by the European Committee for Hyperbaric Medicine. Diving and Hyperbaric Medicine. 2015;**45**(1):42-46

Chapter 4

Postoperative Pain Control Following Cardiac Implantable Electronic Device Implantation

Peter Magnusson, Jo Ann LeQuang and Joseph V. Pergolizzi

Abstract

Postoperative pain following cardiac implantable electronic device (CIED) surgery may not always be adequately treated. The postoperative pain trajectory occurs over several days following the procedure with tenderness and limited arm range of motion lasting for weeks after surgery. Pain control typically commences in the perioperative period while the patient is in the hospital and may continue after discharge; outpatients may be given a prescription and advice for their analgesic regimen. It is not unusual for CIED patients to be discharged a few hours after implantation. While opioids are known as an effective analgesic to manage acute postoperative pain, growing scrutiny on opioid use as well as their side effects and potential risks have limited their use. Opioids may be considered for appropriate patients for a short course of treatment of acute postoperative pain, but other analgesics may likewise be considered.

Keywords: CIED implant, device surgery, ICD implant, ICD implant, implant pain control, implantable cardioverter defibrillator, pacemaker

1. Introduction

Postoperative pain of all types is often under-treated and may lead to chronic postsurgical pain, a centralized painful condition that can be challenging to treat [1]. Reports of postimplant pain can vary. In a survey of pacemaker patients, most patients were satisfied overall with their device and not affected by pain, soreness, or discomfort [2]. Yet in another study, over 40% of surgical patients from a single-center Italian study (n = 235) reported still having mild postsurgical pain at six months [3]. Despite the frequency of device implants for cardiac conditions, there is little study on the incidence, intensity, or duration of pain associated with cardiac implantable electronic device (CIED) implantation.

There is a paucity of literature to inform clinicians about pain management for those undergoing an implantable cardioverter-defibrillator (ICD) or pacemaker implantation. A single-center study from Europe (n = 372) analyzed pain control retrospectively over the course of device implant [4]. The study found about a quarter of patients received analgesia or sedation in advance of surgery. During surgery, all patients received local lidocaine anesthesia. Upon completion of the surgery, less than one-third (31%) were given pain medication or sedated. Using a 0 to 10 numeric rating scale, the highest pain rating during the implantation was 8.

Pain above 5 was reported one, three, six, eight, and 24 hours after surgery, with the most frequently reported pain sites being the surgical incision, shoulder area, and chest region [4].

2. Postoperative pain control

There has been a little systematic study of pain associated with CIED implantation even though, such procedures are increasingly prevalent. Further complicating the subject of postoperative pain control are differences between subcutaneous and transvenous devices and the fact that some implantation procedures are done on an outpatient basis.

2.1 Risk factors for postoperative pain

The BRUISE-CONTROL studies 1 and 2 used a visual analog scale to assess pain in 1308 patients who had a CIED implanted. Using multivariable regression analysis, the following were associated with clinically important postsurgical pain: clinically significant hematoma (odds ratio [OR] 3.8), *de novo* CIED implantation (OR 1.9), female sex (OR 1.6), age < 65 years (OR 1.5), and body mass index <20 (OR 2.1) [5].

In a study of 21 consecutive adult CIED patients (mean age 61 ± 11 years), patients were asked to rate their pain on a 0 to 100 visual analog scale, where 0 was no pain at all and 100 was the worst possible pain imaginable. Patients rate their pain 24 hours after surgery and again at one month postoperatively. At 24 hours postimplant, the mean VAS score was 34 ± 20. Only one patient in the study experienced severe pain, with the rest rating pain as moderate (48%) or mild (48%). Using regression analysis, it was found that the use of intraoperative fentanyl and a longer time spent in the procedure were significant predictors of more intense postoperative pain. The mean VAS score for pain at one month was 19 ± 18 and 17 out of 21 patients rated this pain as "mild" [6].

2.2 Inpatient versus outpatient pain control

Device implantation may be done on an inpatient or outpatient basis, depending on a variety of factors, including patient characteristics, comorbidities, physician preference, geography, patient frailty, and other factors. A retrospective chart review of 415 consecutive primary-prevention ICD patients found that same-day discharge was safe and feasible [7]. However, in real-world clinical practice, many such procedures are performed on inpatients. In a prospective study of 327 *de novo* ICD patients, 40.3% were implanted during acute hospitalization [8]. Of these inpatients, 57.6% were secondary-prevention patients [8]. Predictors of hospitalization include, a more complex device (non-single-chamber device), New York Heart Association (NYHA) class IV symptoms, low diastolic blood pressure, higher blood urea nitrogen levels, and lower hemoglobin [8].

2.3 Subcutaneous ICDs

Subcutaneous ICDs are often implanted under general anesthesia and postoperative pain may be managed with opioid analgesia. However, there is a trend toward moving away from general anesthesia and postoperative opioids to a different type of pain control [9]. Monitored anesthesia care (MAC) has been reported in the literature to be a safe and effective method for subcutaneous ICD implantation [10, 11]. The truncal plane block along with perioperative nonopioid analgesics is being considered and appears feasible and effective [12]. A study of 91 consecutive patients undergoing subcutaneous ICD implantation at 10 centers found ultrasound-guided serratus anterior plane block was effective for anesthesia during the procedure and postoperative analgesia [13].

The Subcutaneous Defibrillator and Send Home (DASH) study investigated the feasibility and safety of subcutaneous ICD implant in patients (mean age 47 ± 14 years) discharged on the same day [14]. In total, 49 patients were enrolled and all were discharged following the surgery without staying overnight at the hospital. The protocol called for preoperative acetaminophen 975 mg and oxycodone 10 mg, local bupivacaine during the surgery, and limited fixed-dose combination oral analgesic of oxycodone plus acetaminophen (5/325 mg) after surgery, every 6 hours as needed. Using a 0 to 10 numerical pain rating scale, severe pain (defined as a score ≥ 8) occurred in 14.3% of patients on the day of surgery, 14.3% on postoperative day 1, and 8.2% of patients on a postoperative day 3 [14].

In a study of 104 adult patients undergoing subcutaneous ICD implantation, 69% were administered intraprocedural liposomal bupivacaine but there were no statistically significant differences between those who received bupivacaine and those who did not in terms of inpatient opioid consumption, outpatient opioid prescriptions, or overall opioid consumption in the postoperative period [15]. Similar findings were observed in a study of liposomal bupivacaine in knee arthroplasty [16].

In a study of opioid use following CIED implantations, patients who underwent subcutaneous ICD implantation were more likely to be prescribed opioids than those implanted with transvenous devices (25% vs. 20%) [17]. In a retrospective single-center study of structured interviews with female patients who were implanted with a subcutaneous ICD (mean time since implant 4.6 ± 3.1 years) 54% said their postsurgical pain was worse than they expected [18]. About half (44%) said that they experienced daily discomfort with their bra and the implanted device [18]. Thus, while postoperative pain can be managed following subcutaneous ICD implant, there are important gaps to be recognized in how pain is treated. In particular, patients should be advised about the nature, duration, and intensity of pain anticipated and provided with an analgesic regimen with specific instructions.

2.4 Device revision

ICDs and other CIEDs require replacement upon battery depletion, and the incidence of any type of complication within 45 days of device revision is 4.3% [19]. Device infections are more common for ICD and CRT-D system revisions than initial implants (2.9% and 3.9% for revisions, respectively, and 1.6% for both ICD and CRT-D *de novo* systems) [20]. It should be noted in this context that a CRT-D system is a more complicated device than a transvenous ICD, even a dual-chamber ICD, and requires a left-ventricular lead. This risk for infection may be cumulative with subsequent device revisions; in fact, each intervention at the same implant site appears to double the risk for infection [21]. There are no studies, comparing postoperative pain intensity or characteristics of initial and revised procedures. Since up to 40% of ICD procedures involve a generator replacement [22], this represents a significant knowledge gap.

In an analysis of opioid prescribing for CIED implantation, patients undergoing device upgrades and generator change-outs were less likely to receive opioids than those getting a *de novo* implant (18.3%, 11.6%, and 20%, respectively) [17].

2.5 Special populations

2.5.1 Pediatric

The number of pediatric device patients is a relatively small subset of the device population, but babies, as well as children and adolescents, may be recipients of CIEDs. Nerve blocks have been effectively used in pediatric patients undergoing implantation of a subcutaneous ICD [23]. In this case series of 10 patients, the combination of bilateral parasternal blocks with a left erector spinae plane block provided good pain control. Pectoral nerve blocks have been shown to reduce perioperative anesthetic requirements and postoperative pain in children undergoing transvenous ICD implantation [24].

2.5.2 Women

A study of 180 men and 60 women, who had a *de novo* ICD implantation, found that women were statistically significantly more likely to be younger and less likely to be married or have a history of coronary artery disease than men [25]. However, women had lower functional status, reported more intense pain, and had more sleep problems than men. Men and women were similar in terms of symptoms of anxiety and depression [25]. A study of 179 consecutive ICD outpatients (mean age 60.5 ± 15.9 years) found women reported significantly more intense pain than men [26].

Women have been historically under-represented in ICD clinical trials and historically were sometimes overlooked in consideration for ICD implantation. In a retrospective study of 5156 outpatients with an ejection fraction ≤35%, 25.0% of women had received an ICD compared to 36.3% men ($p < 0.01$) [27]. In an observational study based on Get with the Guidelines-Heart Failure Program, 21,059 patients with an ejection fraction ≤35%, were evaluated in the time frame from 2011 to 2014. During this time, women were less likely to be counseled about ICD therapy than men (19.3% vs. 24.6%, $p < 0.001$) [28]. It may be that women who receive ICDs are not adequately counseled about what to expect from surgery or treated for pain.

2.5.3 Overweight

Studies suggest that obese patients, defined as a body mass index >30 kg/m^2, are at an elevated risk for inappropriate shock and failed defibrillation testing when a subcutaneous device is implanted [29, 30]. Electrocardiographic testing before implant and appropriate patient selection may reduce such risks [10]. It is unknown whether obese patients experience more pain or more intense pain than normal-weight patients.

2.5.4 Racial/ethnic groups

In a retrospective analysis of 5156 outpatients with an ejection fraction ≤35%, 28.0% of Black compared to 33.2% of White patients had an ICD, $p = 0.02$ [27]. Although this difference was statistically significant, it was less pronounced than sex-based differences in ICD implantation, where men were more likely to receive an ICD than women [27]. Since Blacks Americans are less likely to have health insurance than Whites, it might be speculated that part of this difference can be traced back to differences in health coverage. However, a study from the United Kingdom found that despite free, universal healthcare, there were racial disparities in ICD implantations; ICDs in the United Kingdom were significantly more likely to be implanted in White than South Indian residents [31]. Although the population of Caucasians in the area of Leicestershire was 77.7% and South Asians made up 15.9% of the population, 91.9% of all ICDs in that areas were implanted in Caucasians compared to 8.1% South Asians. These differences persisted for primary- and secondary-prevention patients although the gap between Caucasians and South Asians was even wider for secondary-prevention treatment [31]. It is unclear, why this marked difference occurs. The lower rate of Black patients for ICD therapy is particularly concerning because Blacks are at greater risk than Whites for sudden cardiac death [32]. However, in the United States, Blacks also had a higher ICD refusal rate than other groups when ICD therapy was presented to them as a consideration [32]. Among patients who are at higher risk of sudden cardiac death, Blacks had significantly less probability of getting an ICD [33].

2.5.5 Geriatric

Advanced age and frailty have been associated with less-frequent use of ICD systems and indications require the patient have a reasonable expectation to live at least one more year after device implant [34]. This life expectancy requirement is not always taken into account. In a survey of 386 physicians who refer selected patients for possible ICD implantation, 23% said that they do not consider life expectancy and 13% have knowingly referred patients with a life expectancy of under one year [35]. However, there is no specific age cutoff for ICD indications. More than 40% of all first implants of ICD systems occur in patients over the age of 70, and *de novo* patients over age 80 are not uncommon [36]. Biological age may be more important than chronological age in this regard [37].

Postsurgical pain in geriatric device patients is not well studied; indeed, elderly patients are often under-represented in clinical trials, if they are included at all. In a study of 150,264 primary-prevention patients, there were significantly more adverse events in the oldest patients (4.5% in those ≥80 years) compared to the youngest group (2.8% in those <65 years) [38]. This rate of adverse events plateaued at about 4.5% at age 80 and beyond. Comorbid conditions were stronger predictors for complications than age [38]. However, the proportions of older and younger patients who specifically experienced pain were not reported.

The control of postsurgical pain in geriatric patients can be challenging due to comorbid conditions, concurrent drug therapies (polypharmacy), and age-related pharmacokinetic and pharmacodynamic alterations [39]. Pain assessment maybe even more challenging in elderly patients with impaired communication skills or cognitive deficits. Because elderly patients may get benefit from ICD therapy and may have special limitations with respect to pain therapy, further study is much needed.

2.6 Opioid considerations

Opioids have come under increasing scrutiny as routine analgesics since the Centers for Disease Control and Prevention (CDC) published guidance to limit their use because of growing concerns for their risks, opioid-associated side effects, and opioid use disorder (OUD). In addition, opioids may increase the risk of atrial fibrillation or other arrhythmias [40]. Nevertheless, opioids are effective analgesic agents and are often used for appropriate patients under clinical supervision to manage the acute pain associated with surgery.

In a retrospective analysis of all CIED procedures done at the three Mayo Clinics in Minnesota, Arizona, and Florida, from 2010 to early 2018, opioids were prescribed to 20.2% of the 16,517 patients (mean age 70 ± 15 years) after device implantation. Of this group, 80% were opioid naïve. Of the opioid-naïve patients, 9.4% refilled their opioid prescription at least once and 38.8% of patients received >200 oral morphine equivalents (ME) [17]. The mean amount of ME prescribed was 243 ± 346 overall. Opioid-experienced patients were prescribed significantly more opioids than opioid-naïve patients with 335 ME compared to 219 ME for the opioid-naïve patients ($p < 0.001$) [17].

Opioids are associated with many well-known side effects, including nausea, somnolence, mental fogginess, pruritus, and constipation [41]. In most cases, these side effects are mild to moderate although they can in some instances be severe and even treatment-limiting. A short course of postsurgical opioids typically does not result in treatment-limiting side effects, although some patients find opioid analgesics unpleasant. In a study of 250 surgical inpatients, who had a variety of different types of surgery, 25% of those who had received some form of analgesic reported having side effects, although 90% said that they were satisfied with the pain control medications they were administered [42].

2.7 Clinical strategies: Preoperative, perioperative, postoperative

Although this chapter deals with postoperative pain control following device implant, it is difficult to discuss pain management isolated to the specific postoperative period without describing preoperative and perioperative techniques, which can affect the pain experienced by the patient when the procedure has ended and the patient enters recovery.

2.7.1 Preoperative

The implant of an ICD or any CIED can be associated with severe acute pain. The pain is most intense immediately after the implant procedure and diminished gradually over the next few days as the implant site heals. Postoperative pain should be managed with preoperative, perioperative, and postoperative strategies. In discussing the device implant with the patient, the clinical team should educate the patient on pain control goals and available options with their risks and benefits. It is important to manage the patient's expectations because complete pain eradication is likely not possible. It has been found that oral gabapentin (600–1200 mg) or pregabalin (150–300 mg) administered an hour or two before surgery can reduce postsurgical opioid consumption [43, 44]. Likewise, oral celecoxib (200–400 mg) 30 minutes to 1 hour before surgery can likewise diminish the need for postoperative opioids [43, 45]. Note that the individual patient must be considered in any analgesic regimen; nonsteroidal anti-inflammatory drugs such as celecoxib may be contraindicated in certain cardiology patients.

A structured plan to help to reduce the pain associated with CIED implantation and other related procedures, such as catheter ablation, could significantly reduce pain up to 8–24 hours after the procedure [46]. The elements of such programs include patient education, regular pain assessments, analgesic protocols, and prompt referrals to pain specialists if the pain becomes severe or cannot be managed.

It is concerning that many device patients do not receive any preoperative analgesics. In a study from Croatia, it was found that 75% of patients undergoing CIED implantation received no preoperative pain medications at all [4].

2.7.2 Perioperative

Perioperative pain control is typically managed by local medications and/or regional anesthesia [4]. Proper device placement in the fascia and good hemostasis during the procedure may reduce pain following the operation. Liposomal bupivacaine extended-release formulation may provide good anesthetic infiltration with an effect that can last up to 72 hours [47]. In some cases, general anesthesia is used but truncal plane blocks may also provide adequate anesthesia for difficult procedures or those involving a subcutaneous device [12]. For conventional ICDs and devices with transvenous lead systems, local anesthetic infiltration is probably adequate, but sometimes cervical or pectoral nerve block may be employed [48, 49]. Intravenous ketamine is not recommended because of the potential for myoclonus, which can interfere with device function and cause double-counting [17].

2.7.3 Postoperative

Following surgery, the patient may get benefit from oral analgesics to manage acute pain. Opioid analgesics may be considered for a short course in appropriate patients. A great concern about the use of opioids in any patient is the potential for OUD. Risk stratification tools exist that can help to determine which patients may be at elevated risk for opioid misuse and abuse [50] (see **Table 1**). Opioid overdose may result in potentially life-threatening respiratory depression; naloxone is a rapid-acting rescue drug. Patients taking opioids following CIED implantation may benefit from a prescription for naloxone and the family or caregivers should be trained in how to administer it in an emergency.

In a single-center retrospective study from Croatia (n = 372), 31% of patients being implanted with an ICD received pain medication following surgery; the highest intensity pain recorded in this study was 8 on a 0 to 10 scale [4]. The most frequently prescribed medications in this study were fixed-dose combination oral tramadol and acetaminophen 37.5/325 mg (29%), diazepam 5 mg (17%), tramadol 5 mg monotherapy (16%), and acetaminophen monotherapy

Instruments	Description	Optimal use	Comments
4-A	Observations Analgesia, activities of daily living, adverse events, aberrant drug-taking behaviors	Suitable for ongoing opioid therapy	Not validated
Diagnosis, Intractability, Risk, and Efficacy Inventory (DIRE)	Scoring system	More suitable for long-term therapy or ongoing therapy	Clinician does assessment
Opioid Risk Tool	Clinician-guided questionnaire-based interview; stratifies low, medium, and high risk for aberrant drug-taking behaviors	May be used before start of opioid therapy	High degree of sensitivity and specificity
Pain Medication Questionnaire (PMQ)	Questionnaire	Designed for chronic pain patients	Validated translated versions available
Screener and Opioid Assessment for Patients with Pain-Revised (SOAPP-R)	Questionnaire	To identify those at low risk of OUD	Validated translated versions available

Table 1.
While there is no consensus as to the best opioid-screening tool, a variety of validated instruments exist [51–53]. In place of an assessment tool, a clinical interview with the patient may be conducted to assess past drug experiences, familial history of substance use disorders, and attitudes about pain control. Note that these tools are often used in the setting of long-term opioid therapy, rather than short-term postoperative use.

500 mg (12%) [4]. It should be noted that in this study 69% of patients received no postoperative analgesic medications at all [4]. This strongly suggests that many CIED patients have poorly controlled pain after surgery. Of course, postoperative pain control may be inadequate for many types of surgery. In USA survey of surgical inpatients, who had a variety of procedures, about 80% reported they suffered pain following surgery with 86% of them ranking this pain as "moderate" to "severe" [42]. Perhaps most important is that pain was reported to occur more frequently after discharge than before [42]. Patients may not always know what to expect and some may accept moderate to severe postoperative pain following surgery, not knowing that postoperative pain can often be safely and effectively managed.

An important analgesic strategy involves a combination of multimodal analgesia. Multimodal analgesia is based on the use of two or more analgesics with different mechanisms of action to offer a synergistic benefit to patients. Some fixed-dose combination products offer oral acetaminophen plus, a small amount of opioid, such as oxycodone, in a single oral dose. Adjuvant agents may also be helpful such as gabapentin or pregabalin to help with a neuropathic component to postsurgical pain.

A challenge in pain management following implant is the fact that most device patients do not spend prolonged periods of time in the hospital. Most CIED patients are discharged home shortly after surgery, whether they are outpatients or spend the night in the hospital. Thus, most device patients must manage the longest duration of their postsurgical pain at home. For this reason, patients and their families or caregivers must be educated about the pain medications they are to take, the appropriate doses and timing, and the risks as well as the benefits of these medications. Following transvenous device implant, patients should be educated about arm movements to prevent capsulitis ("frozen shoulder") [54].

3. Conclusions

With millions of device patients around the world, it is important to develop good guidance in terms of how to manage postoperative pain in these patients. Most postoperative pain is moderate to severe but has a predictable trajectory in which the pain is most intense immediately after surgery and diminished day over day over the course of several days. A good strategy for pain control for CIED patients is to consider managing pain perioperatively and then offer the patient postoperative counseling for pain management at home along with appropriate analgesics. For appropriate patients, a short course of opioid analgesics may be appropriate but other nonopioid agents may be considered as well. Subcutaneous ICD implantation is likely associated with more severe or longer-duration postoperative pain although there are no specific head-to-head comparative pain studies. Barring complications, device patients recover over the course of days and weeks and should need analgesia only for a short duration of time.

Conflict of interest

Peter Magnusson has received speaker's fees or grants from Abbott, Alnylam, Amicus Therapeutics, AstraZeneca, Bayer, BMS, Boehringer-Ingelheim, Coala Life, Internetmedicin, Lilly, MSD, Novo Nordisk, Octopus Medical, Orion Pharma, Pfizer, Sanofi, Vifor Pharma, and Zoll.

Jo Ann LeQuang has no disclosures.

Joseph Pergolizzi is a consultant/speaker, owner, or researcher for Spirify, US World Meds, Salix, Enalare, Scilex, Pfizer, Lilly, Teva, Taketa, Regeneron, Grünenthal, Neumentum, NativeCardio, BDSI, and Bridge Therapeutics.

Author details

Peter Magnusson[1,2,3], Jo Ann LeQuang[4*] and Joseph V. Pergolizzi[4]

1 Department of Caring Services, Faculty of Health and Occupational Studies, University of Gävle, Gävle, Sweden

2 Centre for Research and Development, Uppsala University/Region Gävleborg, Gävle, Sweden

3 Cardiology Research Unit, Department of Medicine, Solna, Karolinska Institutet, Stockholm, Sweden

4 NEMA Research, Inc., Naples, Florida, United States of America

*Address all correspondence to: joannlequang@gmail.com

References

[1] Lesin M, Domazet Bugarin J, Puljak L. Factors associated with postoperative pain and analgesic consumption in ophthalmic surgery: A systematic review. Survey of Ophthalmology. 2015;**60**(3):196-203

[2] Magnusson P, Liv P. Living with a pacemaker: Patient-reported outcome of a pacemaker system. BMC Cardiovascular Disorders. 2018;**18**(1): 110

[3] Sansone P, Pace MC, Passavanti MB, Pota V, Colella U, Aurilio C. Epidemiology and incidence of acute and chronic Post-Surgical pain. Annali Italiani di Chirurgia. 2015;**86**(4):285-292

[4] Biocic M, Vidosevic D, Boric M, Boric T, Giunio L, Fabijanic D, et al. Anesthesia and perioperative pain management during cardiac electronic device implantation. Journal of Pain Research. 2017;**10**:927-932

[5] Nair GM, Birnie DH, Sumner GL, Krahn AD, Healey JS, Nery PB, et al. Post-operative pain following cardiac implantable electronic device implantation: Insights from the BRUISE CONTROL trials. Europace. 2021;**23**(5): 748-756

[6] Bollmann A, Marx A, Sathavorn C, Mera F, DeLurgio D, Walter PF, et al. Patient discomfort following pectoral defibrillator implantation using conscious sedation. Pacing and Clinical Electrophysiology. 1999;**22**(1 Pt 2): 212-215

[7] Darda S, Khouri Y, Gorges R, Al Samara M, Jain SK, Daccarett M, et al. Feasibility and safety of same-day discharge after implantable cardioverter defibrillator placement for primary prevention. Pacing and Clinical Electrophysiology. 2013;**36**(7):885-891

[8] Nishimura M, Sab S, Birgersdotter-Green U, Krummen D, Schricker A, Raissi F, et al. Reasons for and predictors of acute hospitalization versus elective outpatient implantable cardioverter-defibrillator implantation and subsequent differential clinical outcomes. Journal of Interventional Cardiac Electrophysiology: An International Journal of Arrhythmias and Pacing. 2017;**50**(1):85-93

[9] Afzal MR, Okabe T, Hsu K, Cook S, Koppert T, Weiss R. How to minimize peri-procedural complications during subcutaneous defibrillator implant? Expert Review of Cardiovascular Therapy. 2020;**18**(7):427-434

[10] Vedachalam S, Cook S, Koppert T, Okabe T, Weiss R, Afzal MR. Approaches to minimizing periprocedural complications during subcutaneous implantable cardioverter-defibrillator placement. The Journal of Innovations in Cardiac Rhythm Management. 2020;**11**(5):4100-4105

[11] Afzal MR, Okabe T, Koppert T, Tyler J, Houmsse M, Augostini RS, et al. Implantation of subcutaneous defibrillator is feasible and safe with monitored anesthesia care. Pacing and Clinical Electrophysiology. 2019;**42**(12): 1552-1557

[12] Miller MA, Garg J, Salter B, Brouwer TF, Mittnacht AJ, Montgomery ML, et al. Feasibility of subcutaneous implantable cardioverter-defibrillator implantation with opioid sparing truncal plane blocks and deep sedation. Journal of Cardiovascular Electrophysiology. 2019;**30**(1):141-148

[13] Ziacchi M, Bisignani G, Palmisano P, Scalone A, Martignani C, Elvira Mocavero P, et al. Serratus anterior plane block in subcutaneous implantable cardioverter defibrillator implantation: A case-control analysis. Journal of Cardiovascular Electrophysiology. 2020;**31**(1):144-149

[14] Okabe T, Miller A, Koppert T, Cavalcanti R, Alcivar-Franco D, Osei J, et al. Feasibility and safety of same day subcutaneous defibrillator implantation and send home (DASH) strategy. Journal of Interventional Cardiac Electrophysiology: An International Journal of Arrhythmias and Pacing. 2020;**57**(2):311-318

[15] Lee JZ, Glasgow AE, Habermann EB, Scott L, Shen WK, Kusumoto FM, et al. Liposomal bupivacaine during subcutaneous implantable cardioverter defibrillator implantation for pain management. Pacing and Clinical Electrophysiology. 2021;**44**(3):513-518

[16] Pichler L, Poeran J, Zubizarreta N, Cozowicz C, Sun EC, Mazumdar M, et al. Liposomal Bupivacaine does not reduce inpatient opioid prescription or related complications after knee arthroplasty: A database analysis. Anesthesiology. 2018;**129**(4):689-699

[17] Lee JZ, Pasha AK, Glasgow AE, Habermann EB, Kusumoto FM, McLeod CJ, et al. Postoperative opioid prescription patterns and new opioid refills following cardiac implantable electronic device procedures. Heart Rhythm. 2019;**16**(12):1841-1848

[18] van der Stuijt W, Quast ABE, Baalman SWE, Olde Nordkamp LRA, Wilde AAM, Knops RE. Improving the care for female subcutaneous ICD patients: A qualitative study of gender-specific issues. International Journal of Cardiology. 2020;**317**:91-95

[19] Krahn AD, Lee DS, Birnie D, Healey JS, Crystal E, Dorian P, et al. Predictors of short-term complications after implantable cardioverter-defibrillator replacement: Results from the Ontario ICD database. Circulation. Arrhythmia and Electrophysiology. 2011;**4**(2):136-142

[20] Clémenty N, Carion PL, Léotoing L, Lamarsalle L, Wilquin-Bequet F, Brown B, et al. Infections and associated costs following cardiovascular implantable electronic device implantations: A nationwide cohort study. EP Europace. 2018;**20**(12): 1974-1980

[21] Arana-Rueda E, Pedrote A, Frutos-López M, Acosta J, Jauregui B, García-Riesco L, et al. Repeated procedures at the generator pocket are a determinant of implantable cardioverter-defibrillator infection. Clinical Cardiology. 2017;**40**(10): 892-898

[22] Hammill SC, Kremers MS, Stevenson LW, Heidenreich PA, Lang CM, Curtis JP, et al. Review of the registry's fourth year, incorporating lead data and pediatric ICD procedures, and use as a National performance measure. Heart Rhythm. 2010;**7**(9): 1340-1345

[23] Koller MP, Cortez D, Kim TW. Nerve blocks for postoperative pain management in children receiving a subcutaneous implantable cardioverter-defibrillator: A case series. A&A Practice. 2020;**14**(13):e01351

[24] Yang JK, Char DS, Motonaga KS, Navaratnam M, Dubin AM, Trela A, et al. Pectoral nerve blocks decrease postoperative pain and opioid use after pacemaker or implantable cardioverter-defibrillator placement in children. Heart Rhythm. 2020;**17**(8):1346-1353

[25] Smith G, Dunbar SB, Valderrama AL, Viswanathan B. Gender differences in implantable cardioverter-defibrillator patients at the time of insertion. Progress in Cardiovascular Nursing. 2006;**21**(2):76-82

[26] Rahmawati A, Chishaki A, Sawatari H, Tsuchihashi-Makaya M, Ohtsuka Y, Nakai M, et al. Gender disparities in quality of life and psychological disturbance in patients with implantable cardioverter-

defibrillators. Circulation Journal. 2013;**77**(5):1158-1165

[27] Johnson AE, Adhikari S, Althouse AD, Thoma F, Marroquin OC, Koscumb S, et al. Persistent sex disparities in implantable cardioverter-defibrillator therapy. Pacing and Clinical Electrophysiology. 2018;**41**(9): 1150-1157

[28] Hess PL, Hernandez AF, Bhatt DL, Hellkamp AS, Yancy CW, Schwamm LH, et al. Sex and race/ethnicity differences in implantable cardioverter-defibrillator counseling and use among patients hospitalized with heart failure: Findings from the Get With The Guidelines-Heart Failure Program. Circulation. 2016;**134**(7):517-526

[29] Amin AK, Gold MR, Burke MC, Knight BP, Rajjoub MR, Duffy E, et al. Factors associated with high-voltage impedance and subcutaneous implantable defibrillator ventricular fibrillation conversion success. Circulation. Arrhythmia and Electrophysiology. 2019;**12**(4):e006665

[30] Frankel DS, Burke MC, Callans DJ, Stivland TM, Duffy E, Epstein AE. Impact of body mass index on safety and efficacy of the subcutaneous implantable cardioverter-defibrillator. JACC: Clinical Electrophysiology. 2018;**4**(5):652-659

[31] Mistry A, Vali Z, Sidhu B, Budgeon C, Yuyun MF, Pooranachandran V, et al. Disparity in implantable cardioverter defibrillator therapy among minority South Asians in the United Kingdom. Heart. 2020;**106**(9):671-676

[32] Thomas KL, Sullivan LT 2nd, Al-Khatib SM, LaPointe NA, Sears S, Kosinski AS, et al. Videos to reduce racial disparities in ICD therapy Via Innovative Designs (VIVID) trial: Rational, design and methodology. American Heart Journal. 2020;**220**:59-67

[33] Thomas KL, Al-Khatib SM, Kelsey RC 2nd, Bush H, Brosius L, Velazquez EJ, et al. Racial disparity in the utilization of implantable-cardioverter defibrillators among patients with prior myocardial infarction and an ejection fraction of <or=35%. The American Journal of Cardiology. 2007;**100**(6):924-929

[34] Munir MB, Alqahtani F, Aljohani S, Bhirud A, Modi S, Alkhouli M. Trends and predictors of implantable cardioverter defibrillator implantation after sudden cardiac arrest: Insight from the national inpatient sample. Pacing and Clinical Electrophysiology. 2018;**41**(3):229-237

[35] Dewland TA, Hsu JC, Castellanos JM, Smith LM, Marcus GM. Consideration of patient age and life expectancy in implantable cardioverter-defibrillator referral. American Heart Journal. 2013;**166**(1):164-170

[36] Epstein AE, Kay GN, Plumb VJ, McElderry HT, Doppalapudi H, Yamada T, et al. Implantable cardioverter-defibrillator prescription in the elderly. Heart Rhythm. 2009;**6**(8): 1136-1143

[37] Barra S, Providência R, Paiva L, Heck P, Agarwal S. Implantable cardioverter-defibrillators in the elderly: Rationale and specific age-related considerations. EP Europace. 2015;**17**(2):174-186

[38] Tsai V, Goldstein MK, Hsia HH, Wang Y, Curtis J, Heidenreich PA. Influence of age on perioperative complications among patients undergoing implantable cardioverter-defibrillators for primary prevention in the United States. Circulation. Cardiovascular Quality and Outcomes. 2011;**4**(5):549-556

[39] Aubrun F, Marmion F. The elderly patient and postoperative pain treatment. Best Practice & Research Clinical Anaesthesiology. 2007;**21**(1): 109-127

[40] Behzadi M, Joukar S, Beik A. Opioids and cardiac arrhythmia: A literature review. Medical Principles and Practice. 2018;**27**(5):401-414

[41] Benyamin R, Trescot AM, Datta S, Buenaventura R, Adlaka R, Sehgal N, et al. Opioid complications and side effects. Pain Physician. 2008;**11** (2 Suppl):S105-S120

[42] Apfelbaum JL, Chen C, Mehta SS, Gan TJ. Postoperative pain experience: results from a national survey suggest postoperative pain continues to be undermanaged. Anesthesia and Analgesia. 2003;**97**(2):534-540 table of contents

[43] Chou R, Gordon DB, de Leon-Casasola OA, Rosenberg JM, Bickler S, Brennan T, et al. Management of Postoperative Pain: A Clinical Practice Guideline From the American Pain Society, the American Society of Regional Anesthesia and Pain Medicine, and the American Society of Anesthesiologists' Committee on Regional Anesthesia, Executive Committee, and Administrative Council. The Journal of Pain. 2016; **17**(2):131-157

[44] Agarwal A, Gautam S, Gupta D, Agarwal S, Singh PK, Singh U. Evaluation of a single preoperative dose of pregabalin for attenuation of postoperative pain after laparoscopic cholecystectomy. British Journal of Anaesthesia. 2008;**101**(5):700-704

[45] Ekman EF, Wahba M, Ancona F. Analgesic efficacy of perioperative celecoxib in ambulatory arthroscopic knee surgery: A double-blind, placebo-controlled study. Arthroscopy. 2006;**22**(6):635-642

[46] Dörschner M, Bollmann A, Dinov B, Richter S, Döring M, Arya A, et al. Structured pain management reduces patient discomfort after catheter ablation and rhythm device surgery. European Journal of Pain. 2017;**21**(10):1723-1731

[47] Malik O, Kaye AD, Kaye A, Belani K, Urman RD. Emerging roles of liposomal bupivacaine in anesthesia practice. Journal of Anaesthesiology Clinical Pharmacology. 2017;**33**(2): 151-156

[48] Martin R, Dupuis JY, Tetrault JP. Regional anesthesia for pacemaker insertion. Regional Anesthesia. 1989;**14**(2):81-84

[49] Mittnacht AJC, Shariat A, Weiner MM, Malhotra A, Miller MA, Mahajan A, et al. Regional techniques for cardiac and cardiac-related procedures. Journal of Cardiothoracic and Vascular Anesthesia. 2019;**33**(2): 532-546

[50] Oliva EM, Bowe T, Tavakoli S, Martins S, Lewis ET, Paik M, et al. Development and applications of the Veterans Health Administration's Stratification Tool for Opioid Risk Mitigation (STORM) to improve opioid safety and prevent overdose and suicide. Psychological Services. 2017;**14**(1):34-49

[51] Kaye AD, Jones MR, Kaye AM, Ripoll JG, Galan V, Beakley BD, et al. Prescription opioid abuse in chronic pain: An updated review of opioid abuse predictors and strategies to curb opioid abuse: Part 1. Pain Physician. 2017; **20**(2s):S93-s109

[52] Webster LR, Webster RM. Predicting aberrant behaviors in opioid-treated patients: Preliminary validation of the opioid risk tool. Pain Medicine. 2005;**6**(6):432-442

[53] Belgrade MJ, Schamber CD, Lindgren BR. The DIRE score:

Predicting outcomes of opioid prescribing for chronic pain. The Journal of Pain. 2006;7(9):671-681

[54] Naffe A, Iype M, Easo M, McLeroy SD, Pinaga K, Vish N, et al. Appropriateness of sling immobilization to prevent lead displacement after pacemaker/implantable cardioverter-defibrillator implantation. Proceedings (Baylor University. Medical Center). 2009;**22**(1):3-6

Chapter 5

CRT Past, Present, and Future Directions: Toward Intelligent Responders Selection and Optimizing Pacing Modalities

Abdullah Alabdulgader

Abstract

Congestive heart failure (CHF) is a serious health problem affecting all nations of world. Its impact is increasing with increasing individual age. Ventricular dyssynchrony is well known to contribute to pathophysiological deterioration in more than one-third of CHF subjects. The therapeutic choices of CHF witnessed long decades of stagnant periods and a relative paucity of effective treatment. The discovery of the electrical therapy that is capable of reversing ventricular dyssynchrony, in the form of cardiac resynchronization therapy (CRT), is a true revolution in the timeline of CHF management. Despite the early enthusiasm associated with CRT implantations started in 2001, we know from the last two decades' experience that non-responders constitute to nearly 40% of all CRT patients. This chapter is devoted to reviewing the past, present and future of CRT with special attention on better intelligent detection of the electrical substrate responsive to CRT as well as optimizing the choice of CRT subjects using the latest knowledge in electrocardiographic and state-of-art imagining technologies. Novel future directions are discussed with new scientific philosophies capable of optimizing CRT. Promising new implants techniques such as endocardial pacing of the left ventricle, His bundle pacing as well as His-optimized cardiac resynchronization therapy are discussed.

Keywords: cardiac resynchronization therapy (CRT), congestive heart failure (CHF), electrical cardiac devices, left bundle branch block (LBBB), right bundle branch block (RBBB), future directions

1. Introduction

Congestive heart failure (CHF) is one of the most important epidemics in the current human species era affecting 1–2% of adults and around 10% of >70 years old in developed countries. The lifetime risk of developing heart failure is one in five after 40 years of age. In the United States, it costs around $39.2 billion in 2010. Sub group of CHF subjects with reduced ejection fraction and electrical dyssynchrony constitutes a true therapeutic challenge. Therapeutic strategies of this CHF sub group witnessed stagnant periods until electrical therapies were introduced to the world communities where cardiac resynchronization therapy (CRT) became available for clinical use first in 2001. Candidates for CRT are CHF subjects with reduced left ventricular systolic function, QRS duration of >120 ms with left bundle branch (LBB) morphology, and functional classification with NYHA class III–IV. Accumulative knowledge in the last two decades has shown that more than one-third of patients are not responding with lack of echocardiographic reverse remodeling or no improvement in quality of life (QOL). Intelligent CRT subjects selection with multidisciplinary expertise and improved procedural skills and strategies, as well as optimizing post-implant care are the main targets to achieve the improved outcomes for the non-responders. Nowadays, a new CRT imaging techniques and innovative pacing strategies are top priorities for us in CHF electrical therapies arena. This chapter is a journey in the CRT timeline reviewing the past, discussing the current situation, and elaborating in future directions for better psychophysiological well-being of CRT subjects.

2. Applying electrical therapy as medicine to treat human disease

Utilizing electric current to treat human disease is an idea that fascinated humans since antiquity. The electrical discharges produced by torpedo fish were utilized as an efficient natural source for electric shock generation by Hippocrates (460–370 BC), Scribonius Largus, and Galen (129–210 AC). It was prescribed for neurological diseases like headache, arthritis gout pain, and prolapsed anus. In 46 AD Scribonius Largus in his compendium of medical treatments known as *Compositiones* described a novel treatment for headache, where, a living black torpedo is put on the place which is in pain, and results were very encouraging. The electric organ of the electric fish can produce amplitudes ranging from 10 to 860 V with a current of up to 1 A. In cardiac science, electrical stimulation was an attractive choice for incapacitating angina pain. An induction coil with sponge-tipped electrodes was used in 1853 to successfully treat abnormal heart rhythms and angina. Relief of angina pectoris by electrical stimulation of the carotid-sinus nerves was achieved repeatedly [1]. The introduction of coronary artery bypass shortly after this convert the electrical stimulation procedure to obsolete. The most fascinating and valuable incorporation of electric therapy in medicine was in the arena of treating rhythm disturbances, either in bradycardia or tachycardia management The first pacemaker was implanted in a person in 1958 and the first lithium battery was introduced in 1969. The deleterious hemodynamic effects of the left bundle branch block (LBBB) had been appreciated by many intelligent observers in the cardiac communities. About 30% of heart failure subjects with reduced ejection fraction with wide QRS interval in the electrocardiogram, tend to have worse clinical outcome [2, 3]. In addition, intraventricular conduction delay (IVCD) was observed as a pathological finding with multiple hemodynamic derangements, including reduced pulse pressure, impaired diastolic function, and mitral regurgitation of functional origin [4]. Early attempts to address this pathology which demonstrated favorable acute hemodynamics and medium-term functional improvements were observed using biventricular pacing [5, 6]. Multisite Stimulation in Cardiomyopathy (MUSTIC) Trial, published in 2001 was the first large trial demonstrating CRT benefits clinically, where three champers are paced, right atrium, right ventricle, and left ventricle. The first CRT device was implanted in the same year. In an attempt to improve the clinical outcome, 10 other prestigious trials were performed. Those 11 clinical trials constitute the determinants and guidelines dictator for CRT practice nowadays. **Table 1** illustrate the details of the inclusion criteria, comparison, and the significant findings of the most influential CRT trials [14]. Nowadays, the cardiac electrical devices communities are investigating methodologies and techniques to improve

CRT outcomes mainly in the non-responders group. The non-LBBB population is classically thought to be out of the selection criteria for CRT. In spite of that, we believe nowadays that 30–50% of these population will benefit from CRT. With this new knowledge, we should convert the necessity of LBBB criteria as lone evidence for ventricular dyssynchrony, an obsolete. In this chapter we are discussing with detail, an innovative diagnostic modalities to hunt the potential responders for CRT. Visionary insight for future speculations will conclude this CRT scientific journey.

Name	Population (n)	Inclusion	Endpoint	Results
MUSTIC SR	58	III, EF < 35%, QRS ≥ 150	6MWT, QoL, pVO2, hospitalization	CRT-P improved : 6MWT, QOL, pVO2; reduced hospitalization
MIRACLE [7]	228-CRT 25-control	III-IV, EF <35%, QRS ≥130	NYHA class, QoL, pVO2	CRT-P improved: NYHA, pVO2, 6MWT
MIRACLE-ICD	186	II, EF < 35%, QRS ≥ 130	6MWT,QoL, hospitalization	CRT-D improved all from baseline (not ICD)
COMPANION [8]	ICM NICM 1,520	III-IV, EF < 35%, QRS > 120	All-cause mortality or hospitalization	CRT-P/CRT-D; reduced endpoints HR 0.80 (CRT vs medical)
CARE-HR [9]	ICM NICM 813	III-IV, EF < 35%, QRS > 120	All-cause mortality or hospitalization	CRT-P/CRT-D; reduced endpoints HR 0.63
MUSTIC AF	59	III, EF < 35%, QRS ≥200 (paced QRS)	6MWT, QoL, pVO2, hospitalization	CRT-P improved : 6MWT, QOL, pVO2, hospitalization
CONTAK-CD			All-cause death + HF hospitalization, pVO2, 6MWT, NYHA class, QoL, LVEDD, LVEF	CRT-D improved: pVO2, 6MWT; reduced LVEDD and increased LVEF
RAFT [10]	1798	II, III, EF <30%, QRS ≥120	Death from any cause or hospitalization for HF	The addition of CRT to an ICD reduced rates of death and hospitalization for HT
REVERSE [11]	610	I-II, EF <40%, QRS ≥ 120	(i) % worsened by clinical composite endpoint, (ii) LVESVi, (iii) HF hospitalization, (iv) all-cause death	Primary endpoint NS; CRT-P/CRT-D reduced (ii) and (iii) hospitalization but not (iv)
MADIT-CRT [12]	ICM NICM 1820	I-II, EF <30%, QRS ≥ 130	(i) HF event or death, (ii) All-cause death, (iii) LVESV	CRT-D reduced (i) and (iii) but not (ii)
MIRACLE-ICD II [13]	186	II, EF <35%, QRS ≥ 130	VE/CO2, pVO2, NYHA, QOL, 6MWT, LV volumes, LVEF	CRT-D improved: NYHA, VE/CO2; volumes, LVEF

Table 1.
Major clinical trials.

3. The dilemma of intelligent resynchronization therapy subjects selection

The philosophy of resynchronizing the electrical stimulation of both ventricles developed into more mature practice, nowadays. The current CRT guidelines are the product of knowledge of the aforementioned clinical trials (**Table 1**) in addition to the accumulation of personal and institutional expert opinions. The most important organizations contributing most importantly to today's guidelines are: American Heart Association, the American College of Cardiology, Heart Rhythm Society, the Heart Failure Society of America, and the European Society of Cardiology. American criteria to define LBBB as defined by AHA/ACC/HRS are as follows:

- QRS >_120
- Notch-, slurred R in I, aVL, V5, and V6
- Occasional RS pattern in V5–V6
- Absent q in I, V5–V6, and aVL
- R peak time >60 ms in V5 and V6
- Normal R-peak time in V1–V3
- No negative concordance
- Usually discordant ST-T segments

The vast majority of recommendations of those organizations are concordant to each other making class I indications clear for CRT specialists to implement. Class I indications are restricted to the symptomatic patients with LVEF ≤35%, NYHA II-IV, with a QRS duration ≥130 ms despite guideline-directed medical treatment (GDMT) [15]. The most recent guidelines are account for the observations that the greatest benefits are consistently seen in those with a QRS duration >150 ms and LBBB pattern [16–18]. On the other hand, echocardiographic evaluation looking for mechanical dyssynchrony results of the Predictors of Response to CRT (PROSPECT) Trial published in 2008 did not show superiority for CRT outcome for any of the predictors [19]. Accumulation of data in the last two decades demonstrated clearly that the CRT success in electrical resynchrony, mechanical remodeling, and quality of life improvement is not always directly linked to the current selection criteria. Response to CRT seems to be more complex than we thought earlier. Currently, 30–40% of our subjects are non-responders. We recommend extension criteria for CRT subjects selection considering the old criteria of QRS duration >130 ms, LV dysfunction (<35%), and NYHA class II-IV as a guideline with more extensive clinical, pathological, imaging and programming variables to be considered. Critical variables such as global scar burden, scar location, lead position, programmed AV and VV interval, mitral regurgitation, and irreversibly advanced heart failure cases are imperative considerations to improve the outcome [20] Despite the traditional dogma that normal QRS duration is a contraindication for CRT, recent challenging groups suggest that QRS complex <130 ms might benefit from CRT. This response as they describe it, is personalized but having QRS complex <130 ms should not be a reason to withhold the option of CRT in systolic heart failure if no other effective treatment is available [21]. Despite the claim that CRT is under-utilized worldwide, we suggest more wise selections with the advanced criteria for more intelligent selection. Our top priority should be the perfection of patients' choices to optimize benefits from CRT. Adjunction of defibrillator therapy with CRT as primary prevention of SCD is indicated in most CRT patients. For this reason, current guidelines advocate an implant of a CRT-D in eligible patients [9, 12]. Most of the systems we are implanting nowadays are CRT-D. This addition of defibrillator stress more for the need of more intelligent and comprehensive criteria for subjects selection. It is imperative to treat any primary disease before thinking of introducing the choice of CRT. Reversible heart diseases such as myocardial ischemia, arrhythmia (tachycardia-induced cardiomyopathy), or primary valvular heart disease must be treated. When AF is a risk factor, catheter ablation of AF is superior to AV node ablation combined with biventricular pacing. This superiority is increasing with the dramatic improvement in our skills and technology, especially with pulmonary veins cryoablation technique. In the subgroup of patients who received prior pacemaker or ICD with worsening heart functions, an upgrade plan for CRT-D seems appropriate. The majority of patients we are implanting, died without experiencing an appropriate ICD shock. A selection system that is capable of predicting survival in patients who received a CRT-D as primary prevention of SCD, identify a subgroup with a significantly poor prognosis despite a CRT-D, as well as being able to discriminate between patients with a low or high risk for mortality, is highly needed. The predictive HF meta-score is constructed of independent mortality predictors identified in a meta-analysis. Three continuous variables constitute this comprehensive evaluation score. In addition to age, LVEF and eGFR, New York Heart Association (NYHA) functional class; 11 dichotomous variables which give the score true discriminative strength including: male gender, African-American race, diabetes, chronic obstructive pulmonary disease, peripheral vascular disease, ischemic cardiomyopathy, HF admission within 1 year before implantation, past or present atrial fibrillation, wide QRS ($\geq$120 ms), secondary prevention indication, and history of ICD shocks (appropriate and inappropriate) [22]. The authors of this meta-analysis found the HF meta-score, a good predictor for survival and useful to detect a subgroup with a significantly poor prognosis despite a CRT-D. In addition, accumulated medical literature in the last few years pin point other conduction system disorders in addition to the major well-known indication of the LBBB as potential indications for CRT. Those indications were based on evidence derived from sub-analyses from the landmark trials and will be discussed in the next section.

4. Understanding the pathophysiological mechanism for becoming a CRT responder

The presence of intrinsic LV electrical dyssynchrony is considered to be the traditional electrical substrate of CRT. Mechanical inefficiency is the result of inefficient electrical-mechanical coupling ending up with triggering two main important outcomes: first is a hemodynamic disturbance in the form of reduced stroke volume and second structural deformation in the form of a cardiac remodeling process. Biventricular pacing, delivered by a CRT device, by correcting the dyssynchrony can improve both hemodynamic and structural derangements [23]. Studying ventricular activation time (known also as intrinsicoid deflection) and variability in activation sequence and passive conduction properties of normal hearts must be perceived very well for accurate comparison and assessment of ventricular dyssynchrony or other activation disorders [24]. Building on this important consideration, we in pacing communities must remind ourselves always of the fact that biventricular pacing is never physiological. Biventricular pacing induces a stage of dyssynchronous electrical activation, remarkably observed at the level of the LV [25].

But with significant baseline electrical dyssynchrony, biventricular activation can be of benefit. Worsening of ventricular synchrony is expected in cases of little or no electrical dyssynchrony resulting in iatrogenic electrical dyssynchrony [25]. Being able to distinguish between patients that may or may not benefit from CRT, is based on a proper understanding of the true deviation from the normal activation pattern of ventricles and proper establishment of the presence of sufficient baseline electrical dyssynchrony.

Research projects supporting this important understanding in biventricular pacing science are multicenter randomized LESSER-EARTH (cardiac resynchronization therapy in patients with heart failure and a QRS complex <120 ms: the evaluation of resynchronization therapy for heart failure) in addition to ECHO-CRT (echocardiography in cardiac resynchronization therapy) trials. Premature termination of patients with narrow QRS duration was elected due to safety concerns [26, 27].

4.1 LBBB is deficient criteria to diagnose CRT responders

Incorporating LBBB as ECG criteria to anticipate responders to CRT is proved to be deficient criteria in at least one-third of patients [28]. In the current CRT literature, there are multiple 'criteria to define LBBB. Present examples are the American Heart Association/American College of Cardiology/Heart Rhythm Society (AHA/ACC/HRS), the European Society of Cardiology (ESC), and Strauss. Clinical outcomes in terms of remodeling reversal, hospitalization for heart failure, survival rates differ between those classifications, as well as clinical outcomes after CRT. In addition, interpretation of slurring and notching differs according to the format and filtering of the ECG. Positioning of the lateral leads is also an important contributing factor. In addition, interpersonal differences in reading ECG impact the LBBB diagnosis [29]. Significant interobserver, and to a lesser extent, intraobserver variability in the classification of LBBB by the use of the various definitions have been documented. Despite applying specific LBBB criteria, 1 in every 5 or 6 ECG will be classified differently by a different observer. If the same observer is tested, 1 in 10 ECG will be classified differently [30]. This conceivably means that a significant proportion of the scientific publications on CRT is niether mentioned nor nonspecific. It is astonishing to know that QRS morphology was not associated with response to CRT with regard to morbidity and mortality in five randomized key CRT trials constituting meta-analysis of data from 3782 patients (CAREHF [Cardiac Resynchronization in Heart Failure], RAFT [Resynchronization/Defibrillation for Ambulatory Heart Failure Trial], MIRACLE [Multicenter InSync Randomized Clinical Evaluation], MIRACLEICD [Multicenter InSync Randomized Clinical Evaluation—Implantable Cardioverter-Defibrillator], REVERSE [Resynchronization Reverses Remodeling in Systolic Left Ventricular Dysfunction]) [31, 32]. *It is clear at this point that what we are looking to treat with CRT is the dominance of leftward electrical delay, not LBBB.* Subjects classified as having LBBB or non-LBBB may or may not have leftward electrical delay [25].

4.2 How to detect dominant left ward electrical delay (LED)

One of the best diagnostic modalities to diagnose electrical-mechanical coupling mismatch is endocardial electrical activation mapping where 3-dimensional electroanatomical reconstruction contact or noncontact mapping can be evaluated with extreme accuracy. Utilizing this unique diagnostic tool declare that in most patients with LBBB there is a dominant leftward electrical delay [33–35]. The ECG imaging or body surface mapping can display electrical activation sequences noninvasively. This predominant leftward electrical conduction delay is a critical component of the electrical substrate, which is amenable for CRT with expected electrical and mechanical derangements recovery.

4.3 The electrical substrate in Intraventricular conduction delay and CRT

A heterogenous and complex ventricular activation pattern, different from bundle branch pattern, is associated with IVCD. This is thought to be due to electrical disease in combination with the myocardial disease [35, 36]. Subjects with IVCD are known to have LV activation time shorter than LBBB subjects. In addition the latest activation time in IVCD is variable. In IVCD subjects electrical delay is not as advanced but there is evidence of underlying myocardial disease. This results in a less favorable response of CRT in IVCD subjects [33, 35, 37]. Ventricular activation studies displayed electrical conduction disturbance in IVCD similar to LBBB in 20–52% of IVCD subjects [33, 35, 37]. This group of patients has the potential of gaining the best advantage from CRT [3]. In patients with typical LBBB, change to atypical LBBB might be indicative of scar formation after myocardial infarction that may benefit from CRT. National Cardiovascular Data Registry Implantable Cardioverter-Defibrillator (NCDR ICD) registry studied 11,505 CRT patients with non-LBBB, demonstrated that CRT implantation appeared to be associated with better outcomes than did implantable cardioverter-defibrillator (ICD) therapy alone in IVCD patients with a QRS duration of > or =150 ms, but not in patients with QRS duration < 150 ms or RBBB [38].

4.4 The electrical substrate responsive to CRT in RBBB

In right bundle branch block (RBBB) subjects the RV is activated slowly after LV activation. This fact explains convincingly the failure of CRT in RBBB subjects. As a matter of fact conventional CRT induces, rather than resolves, electrical dyssynchrony in RBBB subjects. Preclinical research and computer simulations evaluating the hemodynamic consequences of RBBB failing heart document this state of dyssynchrony in this subset of patients [39, 40]. There was no significant difference in total and regional LV endocardial activation times between RBBB and LBBB patients [34]. This fact is not a contradiction to the fact of dyssynchrony induced by CRT in RBBB. The conclusive statement here is that: RBBB subjects who have concomitantly sufficiently significant coexisting LV conduction delay, CRT will result in hemodynamic improvement [39]. *This is a new era of biventricular pacing where RBBB in the ECG may constitute an indication for CRT.* In the 1960s Rosenbaum et al. intelligently mentioned a new RBBB pattern that he called "RBBB masking LBBB," characterized by a broad slurred R wave in leads I and aVL, together with a left axis deviation [41]. In addition, Tzogias et al. in 2014 found that atypical RBBB(RBBB pattern in lead V1 and absent significant S-wave in the lateral leads I and aVL) might be explained as coexisting left bundle branch delay (bilateral bundle-branch delay) and might suggest possible CRT responders within a group of patients with RBBB [42]. Left hemiblock in the presence of RBBB is another indicator alarming for leftward conduction delay and supporting the decision for biventricular pacing with CRT in RBBB subjects, although heterogeneity of trials data are evident. The heterogeneity of positive outcomes in this group of patients can be explained by the fact that left hemiblock might be a primary conduction system disease with associated dyssynchrony, or by infarction of the proximal left anterior descending coronary artery, where dyssynchrony is absent [43].

4.5 Contribution of CRT to atrioventricular dyssynchrony

Ventricular resynchronization was thought to be the sole target of CRT. Atrioventricular conduction delay represented by prolonged PR interval in the ECG was found to be a potential target for CRT [44]. Consequences of inefficient atrioventricular coupling are elevated LV end-diastolic pressure, diastolic mitral regurgitation, and reduced stroke work. Atrioventricular conduction disturbances are frequent findings in the heart failure population with an increased rate of hospitalization, atrial fibrillation, and mortalities [45]. CRT was found to be associated with worsened outcomes in prolonged PR intervals compared to normal patients in several nonrandomized trials [46, 47]. In contrast, subanalyses in two of the MADIT-CRT trial, investigating CRT effects on patients with non-LBBB and long PR interval, document reduction in the risk of all-cause mortality as well as heart failure hospitalization [48–50]. *In conclusion, our directions now considering differences in methodology, design, and outcome measures in different studies, obviate drawing solid conclusion to decide for atrioventricular dyssynchrony as electrical substrate responsive to CRT.*

5. Response prediction of new echocardiographic mechanical dyssynchrony markers

5.1 Eye balling and time-based mechanical dyssynchrony markers

Accumulation of resynchronization trials knowledge demonstrated clearly that an important proportion of the CRT population is not responding. All-cause mortality combined including heart failure hospitalization, NYHA class, and patient global assessment were used in a heart failure clinical composite score (CCS) in Multicenter InSync Randomized Clinical Evaluation (MIRACLE) and was not able to show improvement in 34% of patients [7, 51]. A special new concern group in today's trials are the non-LBBB subjects. The use of echocardiographic markers before 2008 for this important group was not able to show additive benefit of the use of echocardiographic markers to predict CRT in important landmark trials like PROSPECT (Predictors of Response to Cardiac Resynchronization Therapy), ECHO-CRT, and others [26]. Iatrogenic electropathy has been reported as a possible deleterious effect of biventricular pacing [52]. *New echocardiographic parameters to evaluate ventricular dyssynchrony were made available to provide proper measurement tool for resynchronization therapy* [53, 54]. Two parameters are in clinical use nowadays: first is simple eyeballing to assess the degree of dyssynchrony. The second is more technical demanding based on strain study called strain-based speckle tracking echocardiography (STE). Mechanical dyssynchrony is present when an interventricular mechanical delay of > or = 40 ms and a septal-to-posterior radial peak strain delay of > or = 130 ms assessed with STE-strain curves.

Incorporation of echocardiographic mechanical parameters to evaluate ventricular dyssynchrony contribute significantly to the improvement of the prognostic value of guideline-based patient selection for CRT [54, 55]. Reduction of all-cause mortality was associated with incorporation of the apical rocking and/or septal flash at baseline evaluation for CRT [56, 57]. Incorporation of mechanical dyssynchrony parameters as a selection criterion for CRT was associated with a significant reduction in LV end-systolic pressure in comparison to the old criteria based on QRS duration and morphology alone [55]. Despite those early promising outcome studies, not all non-LBBB with mechanical dyssynchrony have improved outcomes.

Here it is wise to remember that absence of response, especially in the time dyssynchrony-based studies, might be related to a non-electrical disease that is not responding to CRT like myocardial hypocontractility and scaring, which are very frequent pathologies in the heart failure population. Future randomized control trials must consider those important discriminative factors.

5.2 Septal rebound stretch analysis for the prediction of volumetric response to cardiac resynchronization therapy

Utilizing detection of specific wall motion patterns to serve as markers for CRT response is the most recent advance in the investigation toward optimal response prediction for CRT [54, 58–60]. It is promising as a superior ventricular dyssynchrony measure tool compared to timing-based measures. Early septal contraction and delayed lateral wall activation give rise to myocardial stretching of the opposing wall during systole [54, 59, 61, 62]. This stretching is paradoxical systolic LV motion that is not contributing to LV ejection and, will result in waste of energy. This myocardial stretch and the resulting waste of energy can be converted to myocardial shortening when we perform biventricular pacing [58, 63, 64]. Systolic rebound stretch of the septum (SRSsept) refers to the amount of systolic stretching of the septum after initial systolic shortening (**Figure 1**). It is considered as a good indicator to reflect the potential for recovery of LV function with CRT and might be one of the best response indicators for resynchronization therapy [53, 58, 66]. Salden et al. and after their pioneering publication in the strategies to improve the selection of patients without typical LBBB for cardiac resynchronization therapy [67] and in a recent publication, published the first results from the multicenter study that investigated the association of baseline echocardiographic SRSsept with the volumetric response after CRT. They found that SRSsept is independently associated with favorable changes in LVESV post CRT. In addition, they found that for the prediction of volumetric response, assessment of SRSsept implies additional predictive information compared to visual assessment of apical rock alone. For assessment of subjects without strict LBBB criteria, SRSsept is an excellent echocardiographic discriminator to predict response to CRT [65]. We and others recommend incorporation of echocardiographic SRSspet for future prospective validation studies for CRT subjects evaluation.

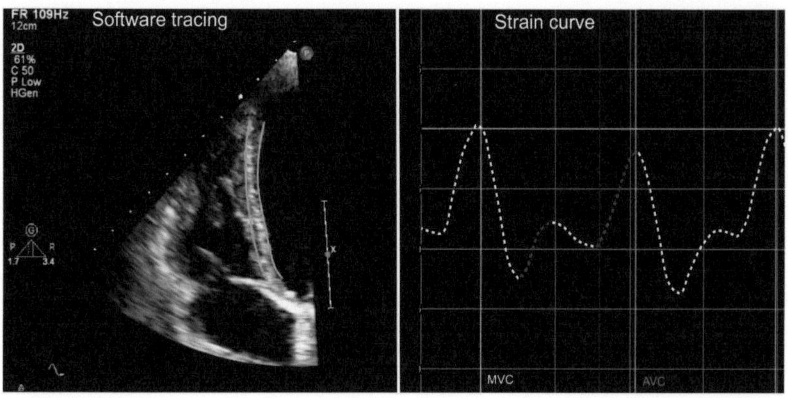

Figure 1.
Septal single wall image acquisition of systolic rebound stretch of the septum (SRSsept)-in red-defined as septal stretching after initial shortening. Speckle tracking echocardiography software was used to deduce strain curves of the focused LV septal wall image. MVC, mitral valve closing; AVC, aortic valve closing [65].

6. Cardiac resynchronization therapy guided by cardiovascular magnetic resonance

Cardiovascular magnetic resonance (CMR) is well known for its unprecedented image quality for cardiac structures as well as for functional assessment of cardiac functions. In addition, it has been introduced to CRT communities as a unique diagnostic tool in differentiating between the various causes of LV dysfunction. CMR is well known to be an excellent evaluating tool for critical factors in the potential response to CRT like a myocardial scar, the total amount of scar (scar burden), and scar location and its relationship to the pacing stimulus. The intricate arrangements of human heart myocardial fibers are a complex anisotropic fiber structure showing longitudinal, circumferential, and oblique layers that form a mechanical link between remote areas of the myocardium [68–71]. Electrically heterogeneous conduction from endocardium to mid-myocardium and epicardium is also a feature of the human heart [72]. Conduction disturbances, superimposing in this inherent anatomical, functional, and electrical heterogeneity of the myocardium is expected to yield multiple areas of dyssynchrony [72, 73]. This finding raises the possibility that deploying an LV lead over a single site of late wall motion may not correct global cardiac dyssynchrony. By the same token, multiple LV leads may be preferable to one LV lead in some patients (**Figure 2**) [74].

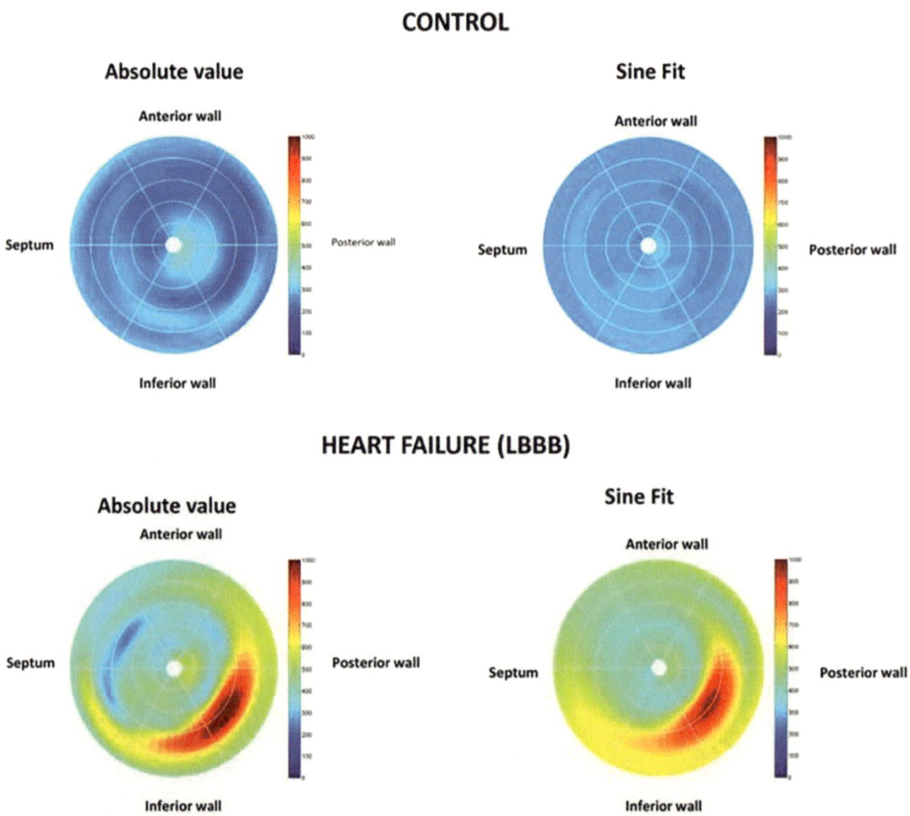

Figure 2.
CMR radial wall mapping illustrating inward wall motion with colors ranging from blue to green and to red. Bull's eye with a homogenous red color throughout denotes complete synchrony, where the bull eye with homogenous blue color denotes complete synchrony. Heterogenous color coding denotes dyssynchrony of radial motion where blue is representing early (global systolic phase) activation and red representing late (global diastolic phase) inward radial wall motion (from Foley et al. [74, 75]).

With its unique discriminative and diagnostic accuracy, CMR has become the gold standard for the in vivo assessment of myocardial scarring. The cutoff point for scar burden, where more is associated with poor response to CRT, is different between different investigators but in general, we consider scar burden less than 15–33% is a potentially good indicator for better response to CRT [76, 77]. Another delicate feature of CMR contribution to CRT management is that CMR can be a fine assessment tool for diagnosing the substrate of heart failure. It is well known that myocardial infarctions can be silent in about one-third of patients and coronary angiography study can be normal after myocardial infarction. In addition, wall motion abnormalities are not equivalent to myocardial ischemia. Unparalleled anatomical imaging, combined with late gadolinium enhancement (LGE)-CMR findings, makes CMR an ideal radiation-free diagnostic tool for the actual heart failure substrate. Scarring in the subendocardial or transmural distribution along arterial territories is typical for infarcted myocardium. Lack of localized myocardial scarring is characteristic of non-ischemic cardiomyopathy or less often, by mid-wall LGE, characterized fibrosis. Myocarditis, sarcoidosis, and arrhythmogenic right ventricular cardiomyopathy are characterized by the patchy distribution of LGE. Amyloidosis and Anderson-Fabry diseases are characterized by diffuse LGE.

7. Cardiac resynchronization therapy guided by computed tomography

Although CMR is an excellent diagnostic tool for evaluating CRT response evaluation, the frequent presence of pacemakers in this group of patients renders its use limited especially in countries where MRI-compatible devices are not available. Non-response to CRT might be caused by factors other than dyssynchrony of electrical activation. Important hidden factors that must gain attention for non-responders are myocardial scar, myocardia hypocontractility, and suboptimal left ventricular (LV) lead location. All of these factors can be investigated with computed tomography (CT). Late iodine enhancement computed tomography (LIE-CT) was found to be an important elegant diagnostic modality in this regard. Théo Pezel et al. investigated CT dyssynchrony measurements for which the LV short-axis images from the multiphase reformatted reconstructions were used [78]. CT dyssynchrony indices used in their investigation were: global and segmental time to maximal wall thickness, global and segmental time to maximal inward wall motion, and time to minimum systolic volume. The dyssynchrony they measured were not the baseline dyssynchrony but the persistent dyssynchrony despite biventricular stimulation. LV lead malpositioning is a serious potentially avoidable reason for non-responders group. Pre-determination of LV lead positioning might be approached by invasive angiogram during implantation and CT coronary angiography. Short axis of the heart is used to determine LV lead final position as anterior, anterolateral, lateral, inferolateral, or inferior. In the long axis of the heart searched positions are basal, mid, or apical. Théo Pezel et al. evaluated concordance of the lead location to regional LV mechanical contraction, where they calculated the mean times to maximal wall thickness and maximal wall motion of each segment using an 8-segment model. Identification of the segment of the myocardium with the latest mean times to either maximal wall thickness or wall motion was determined. Greater global dyssynchrony, as measured by the time to maximal wall thickness, time to peak inward wall motion, and time-to-minimum systolic volume was found between non-responders. Greater segmental dyssynchrony between the anterior and inferior segments, between the inferoseptal and anterolateral segments, and between the anteroseptal and inferolateral segments was found between non-responders. In addition, in the non-responders, the LV lead location was less often concordant with the region of maximal wall thickness (9% vs. 72%, p = .001) [78].

In addition, CT was found to be an appropriate diagnostic tool to follow up the association of LV wall thickness and the ability to reverse LV remodeling and mitral regurgitation improvement after CRT [79].

8. Future directions to optimize cardiac resynchronization therapy

CRT is well known since its inception to be a promising electrical therapeutic device to treat CHF. After more than two decades in clinical use, we know that around 30–40% of CRT subjects do not exhibit any detectable clinical or echocardiographic benefit. As a matter of fact, some of them are deteriorating after resynchronization. For this reason, most of the discussion in this chapter and selected recent literature is devoted to non-responders toward optimizing resynchronization therapy [80, 81]. The special diagnostic tools mentioned earlier in this chapter are to refine our CRT subjects selection especially the subgroup without conspicuous LBBB criteria. Those special diagnostic tools can be still considered as future direction that has been started and in the way for mature applicable understandings in the field of CRT science. *Promising new directions can be classified as new diagnostic tools and new basic knowledge with deeper investigation in the biomechanics of cardiac electromechanical coupling and spatial orientation of the ventricular muscles, as well as ,new advances in implant and resynchronization site.*

8.1 Vectorcardiography guided cardiac resynchronization therapy

Vectorcardiography (VCG) was developed by E. Frank in the mid-1950s. The magnitude and direction of the electrical forces that are generated by the heart are recorded in 3-dimensional information format by means of a continuous series of vectors that form curving lines around a central point. The area under the 3-dimensional QRS complex (QRS area) is reflecting the electrical forces during depolarization and the area under the 3-dimensional T-wave (T area) is reflecting the electrical forces during repolarization. Volumetric response and survival after CRT were thought to be predicted strongly by the QRS area, but also T area and the sum of QRS and T areas (QRST area) [82, 83]. QRS area was also found repeatedly to be superior to QRS duration and morphology as a predictor of CRT response [28, 82, 84, 85]. One retrospective multicenter study displayed that this was true for a cohort of patients that received CRT and also for patients without a Class I indication for CRT according to American guideline recommendations [56] (QRS duration 120–149 ms or non-LBBB) [28]. Only the QRS area in these patients, was significantly associated with all-cause mortality. Reviewing volumetric CRT response, demonstrated that both QRS area and LBBB morphology were associated with an LV end-systolic volume reduction of = or >15 [28]. The advantage of the QRS area is that it is an objective measure and observer-independent parameter, whereas the definition for LBBB is subjective measure and operator-dependent. Variability in the QRS area is less than QRS duration as it is determined by QRS complex amplitude, not the beginning and end of the QRS complex [28]. VCG is not yet commercially available in clinical practice, but the QRS area is a promising non-invasive diagnostic evaluation tool for identifying possible CRT responders.

8.2 Improving our understanding of the biomechanics of cardiac electromechanical coupling and the contribution of spatial orientation of the ventricular muscle band to cardiac pumping functions

Perceiving heart pumping functions as a simple contraction of the bullet-shaped left ventricle is thought nowadays as a misunderstanding which contributes significantly to delaying the successful progress of electrical device treatment for heart failure. The process of contraction and myocardial stretch need more investigation at the cellular, as well as, at gross myocardial fibers orientation level. At the cellular level, electrical activation will trigger mechanical contraction via an intracellular calcium-dependent process known as excitation-contraction coupling. Disturbance of the process of cardiac myocyte intracellular calcium handling is a common feature of heart failure. At the organ scale, pump dysfunction is the end result of mechanical alterations secondary to electrical dyssynchrony in heart failure subjects. A reverse coupling between cardiac mechanics and electrophysiology is also well established. It is commonly referred to as *cardiac mechanoelectric feedback* and is thought to be an important contributor to the increased risk of arrhythmia during pathological conditions that alter regional cardiac wall mechanics, including heart failure. The roles of stretch-activated ion channels and mechanisms that are independent of ionic currents need more investigation. We in the CRT community, are in high demand for new multicellular tissue-scale model systems and experiments to obtain a better understanding of how interactions between electrophysiological and mechanical processes at the cell scale affect ventricular electromechanical interactions at the organ scale in the normal and diseased heart [86]. At a gross level, many observations demand serious investigations considering proper understanding of the mechanics of heart pumping and the true contribution of the spatial orientation of the ventricular muscle band to cardiac pumping functions. Without this knowledge, our understanding and interpretation of ventricular activation and dyssynchrony will be deficient. The existence of right and left ventricles as a continuous muscle band has been proposed [87–90]. The muscle band is organized in special spatial orientation as a helix formed by basal and apical loops. Both ventricular contraction and relaxation controlling the ejection and the filling of ventricles are thought to be affected by this unique arrangement [91, 92]. A deeper investigation of this spatial fibers orientation and the contribution of its activation sequence to cardiac pumping functions in health and disease will improve our therapeutic measures for proper resynchronization of dyssynchronized ventricles. Sengupta PP et al, elaborated in this direction and describe LV as a complex structure in which myofibers are arranged in the form of a left-handed helix in the subepicardium and of a right-handed helix in the subendocardium, while the mid-wall is consisting of circumferential fibers. This type of fibers arrangement allows for myocardial deformation in multiple planes and explains the complexity of the ventricular dyssynchrony process (**Figure 3**) [94]. During LV systole, there is apical counterclockwise rotation and basal clockwise rotation around the LV long axis. During LV diastole, there is Untwisting of the subendocardial layers that occurs during diastole and contribute to diastolic suctioning. Simultaneously, the LV shortens in systole and lengthens in diastole. At this level of understanding, we are confident that the extent of LV mechanical dysfunction is never a matter of one direction of motion or deformation. Future research for resynchronization therapy must consider this basic understanding.

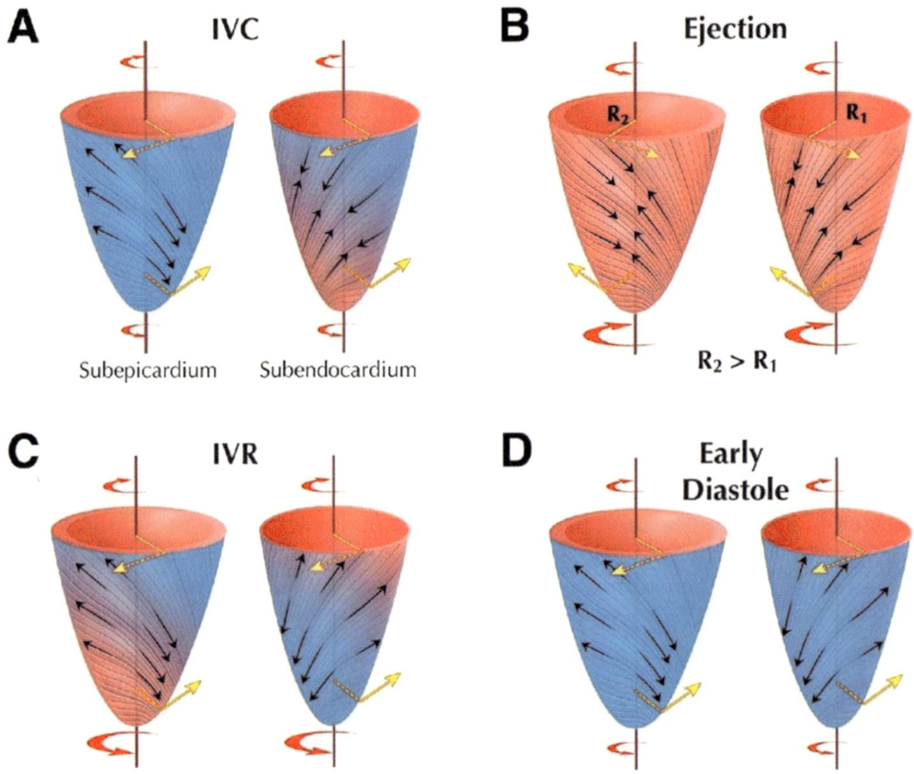

Figure 3.
Twist mechanics of the left ventricle. A period of left ventricular isovolumic contraction (IVC) follows electrical and mechanical activation in the apical subendocardial region, during which (A), the subendocardial myofibers (right-handed helix) shorten with stretching of the subepicardial myofibres (left-handed helix) resulting in clockwise rotation of the apex and counterclockwise rotation of the base. Simultaneous shortening of the subendocardial and subepicardial layers is occurring during ejection (B). The larger arm of the moment of the subepicardial fibers dominates the direction of twist, causing counterclockwise and clockwise rotation of the apex and base, respectively. During isovolumic relaxation (IVR) (C). Subepicardial fibers lengthen from base to apex and subendocardial fibers lengthen from apex to base. In diastole, there is relaxation in both layers, with minimum untwisting (D). Illustration is from Sengupta PP [93].

8.3 Endocardial left ventricular pacing

Challenges of transvenous LV lead implantation including limitations of coronary sinus (CS) anatomy, high LV pacing threshold, and/or phrenic nerve capture, have led to serious efforts to look for better alternatives [94]. As compared to standard epicardial LV pacing, pacing the LV endocardium reflects a more rapid and physiological activation of the left ventricle. Shetty AK et al have identified greater acute hemodynamic improvements with endocardial versus conventional LV pacing [95]. Subjects who demonstrated CRT non-response or known to have LV lead technical difficulties were evaluated in the alternate site cardiac resynchronization study. Endocardial LV lead placement was found to be safe and reported clinical and echocardiographic improvement in two-third of subjects [96]. An important drawback of this new trend of an implant is the need for anticoagulation and the reported few cases of thromboembolic events despite anticoagulation. The endocardial wireless stimulation for CRT (EBR Systems, Sunnyvale, CA, USA) incorporates a pacing system using a small ultrasound-responsive leadless electrode placed onto the LV endocardial surface [97]. The safety and performance of electrodes implanted in the left ventricle study is coming up with encouraging results. A total of 35 patients who had failed conventional CRT implant, underwent successful implant in 97% of the sample [93]. At 6 months, approximately two-thirds of patients demonstrated LV reverse remodeling with improved LVEF ≥5%. LV endocardial pacing seems to be a revolution creator in CRT practice in the present and future.

8.4 His bundle pacing and His-optimized cardiac resynchronization therapy for electrical resynchronization in heart failure

In 1977, Narula et al. reported that the QRS complex may be normalized by pacing the distal His bundle in patients with LBBB [98]. Permanent pacing of the His bundle region to achieve ventricular resynchronizing has been described, with clear clinical advantages over traditional RV apical pacing [99–102]. Medtronic has announced US Food and Drug Administration (FDA) clearance and commercial launch for the SelectSite C304-HIS deflectable catheter system for use in procedures involving His bundle pacing (HBP). The physiologic benefit of permanent His bundle pacing (HBP) is theresult of synchronous electrical and mechanical activation with stimulation of both ventricles through the intrinsic His-Purkinje system. The anatomic site of the conduction disorder seen with BBB is frequently located proximally within the bundle of His, with longitudinal dissociation of the conducting fibers [103, 104]. Overall, it has been reported that approximately three quarters of BBB patients were found to respond with QRS narrowing using HB pacing [103]. Using epicardial electrocardiography (ECG), imaging Arnold et al, demonstrated that HB pacing was superior to biventricular pacing for restoring LV synchrony in selected patients with LBBB [105]. In the presence of distal BBB or the co-existence of IVCD, QRS may not normalize. In patients without complete LBBB correction, Vijayaramanet P et al demonstrated that His-optimized CRT (HOT-CRT) with synchronized LV pacing resulted in significant QRS duration narrowing [106, 107]. In patients with atrioventricular (AV) block in whom fusion with intrinsic His-Purkinje conduction cannot be achieved, HOT-CRT may provide the new therapeutic option. However, it is wise to remember that QRS duration reflects total ventricular activation time which is not always equivalent to a perfect marker of LV synchrony. HOT-CRT was found to be a novel approach to further optimize electrical resynchronization by combining the concept of fused adaptive LV pacing with HBP.

9. Conclusion

CHF is one of the most important epidemics in the current human species era affecting 1–2% of adults and around 10% of >70 years old in developed countries. In addition to its psychophysiological and social burden, the economic impact of CHF on the world nations is Gargantum. Treatment options for CHF witnessed relative stagnation until 2001, where the first electrical device in the form of biventricular pacing to resynchronize the failing desynchronized ventricles, was implanted in 2001. In spite of the early excitement for this type of therapy most international landmark trials reported 30–40% of non-responders. Factors contributing to this large proportion of non-responders are related to scar burden and scar localization to the vicinity of the LV pacing stimulus, hypocontractility, and the degree of pre-implant mechanical dyssynchrony. It was surprising to medical communities to discover that a significant proportion of CHF without LBBB responds to CRT. This chapter is a scientific journey to understand the pathophysiological mechanism to optimize the selection of CRT responders. We confirm that LBBB is deficient criteria for selecting CHF patients for CRT. A spectrum of ventricular conduction disorders that might benefit from CRT, as derived from landmark trials were discussed including IVCD and RBBB. New techniques to detect dominant left ward electrical delay (LED) including endocardial 3-dimensional electroanatomical mapping and ECG imaging or body surface mapping to display electrical activation sequences as well as the elaboration of the best electrical substrate to optimize response to CRT in IVCD, RBBB, and atrioventricular delay are discussed. Determination of pre-implant degree of dyssynchrony is critical as pacing is known to induce more dyssynchrony for mild cases at the baseline with clinical and hemodynamic compromise. For this reason, special attention in this chapter was devoted to new echocardiographic mechanical dyssynchrony markers like eyeballing, septal flash, and time-based mechanical dyssynchrony markers. Systolic septal rebound stretch (SRSsept) was found to be an excellent echocardiographic discriminator to predict response to CRT. Cardiovascular Magnetic Resonance (CMR) was found to be an ideal radiation-free diagnostic tool for the diagnosis of the actual heart failure substrate and accordingly to optimize CRT responders selection. CRM is known to be the gold standard for scar diagnosis but is also considered to be an excellent diagnostic tool for fibrosis, myocarditis, sarcoidosis, arrhythmogenic right ventricular cardiomyopathy, amyloidosis, and Anderson-Fabry disease. Computed tomography is also an excellent tool to diagnose myocardial scar as well as for coronary venous system reconstruction images for optimal LV lead positioning. An innovative future direction for the best outcome of CRT is discussed. The non-invasive nature of vectorcardiography (VCG) with its strong prediction capabilities for volumetric as well as survival indicators after CRT, makes VCG an attractive adjunct diagnostic tool to optimize CRT responders selection. Improving our understanding of the biomechanics of cardiac electromechanical coupling and the contribution of the spatial orientation of the ventricular muscle band to cardiac pumping functions is creating a new visionary approach toward understanding the extent of LV mechanical dysfunction and perfective lead positioning in CRT subjects. New LV lead positions like pacing the LV endocardium reflect a more rapid and physiological activation of the left ventricle with excellent early results. Permanent pacing of the His bundle region to achieve ventricular resynchronizing has been described, with clear clinical advantages over biventricular pacing. Progressive narrowing in QRS duration was documented with HB pacing compared to conventional CRT with the best narrowing was gained with His-optimized cardiac resynchronization therapy (HOT-CRT). This multi-disciplinary approach to optimize CRT response is promising for a better future of resynchronization therapy aiming toward the best possible quality of life for this important group of CHF subjects in the next decades.

Author details

Abdullah Alabdulgader
Prince Sultan Cardiac Center-Alhasa, Hofuf, Saudi Arabia

*Address all correspondence to: kidsecho@yahoo.com

References

[1] Braunwald E, Epstein SE, Glick G, Wechsler AS, Braunwald NS. Relief of angina pectoris by electrical stimulation of the carotid-sinus nerves. The New England Journal of Medicine. 1967;**277**(24):1278-1283. DOI: 10.1056/NEJM196712142772402

[2] Aaronson KD, Schwartz JS, Chen TM, Wong KL, Goin JE, Mancini DM. Development and prospective validation of a clinical index to predict survival in ambulatory patients referred for cardiac transplant evaluation. Circulation. 1997;**95**:2660-2667

[3] Baldasseroni S, Opasich C, Gorini M, et al. Left bundle-branch block is associated with increased 1-year sudden and total mortality rate in 5517 outpatients with congestive heart failure: A report from the Italian network on congestive heart failure. American Heart Journal. 2002;**143**:398-405

[4] Stellbrink C, Nowak B. The importance of being synchronous: On the prognostic value of ventricular conduction delay in heart failure. Journal of the American College of Cardiology. 2002;**40**:2031-2033

[5] Foster AH, Gold MR, McLaughlin JS. Acute hemodynamic effects of atrio-biventricular pacing in humans. The Annals of Thoracic Surgery. 1995;**59**:294-300

[6] Leclercq C, Cazeau S, Le Breton H, et al. Acute hemodynamic effects of biventricular DDD pacing in patients with end-stage heart failure. Journal of the American College of Cardiology. 1998;**32**:1825-1831

[7] Abraham WT, Fisher WG, Smith AL, Delurgio DB, Leon AR, Loh E, et al. Multicenter InSync Randomized Clinical Evaluation. Cardiac resynchronization in chronic heart failure. The New England Journal of Medicine. 2002;**346**:1845-1853

[8] Bristow MR, Saxon LA, Boehmer J, Krueger S, Kass DA, De Marco T, et al. Cardiac-resynchronization therapy with or without an implantable defibrillator in advanced chronic heart failure. The New England Journal of Medicine. 2004;**350**(21):2140-2150. DOI: 10.1056/NEJMoa032423. PMID: 15152059

[9] Cleland JG, Daubert JC, Erdmann E, Freemantle N, Gras D, Kappenberger L, et al. The effect of cardiac resynchronization on morbidity and mortality in heart failure. New England Journal of Medicine. 2005;**352**:1539-1154

[10] Tang ASL, Wells GA, Talajic M, et al. Cardiac-resynchronization therapy for mild-to-moderate heart failure. The New England Journal of Medicine. 2010;**363**:2385-2395. DOI: 10.1056/NEJMoa1009540

[11] Linde C, Abraham WT, Gold MR, St John Sutton M, Ghio S, Daubert C, et al. Randomized trial of cardiac resynchronization in mildly symptomatic heart failure patients and in asymptomatic patients with left ventricular dysfunction and previous heart failure symptoms. Journal of the American College of Cardiology. 2008;**52**(23):1834-1843. DOI: 10.1016/j.jacc.2008.08.027. Epub 2008 Nov 7. PMID: 19038680

[12] Moss AJ, Hall WJ, Cannom DS, Klein H, Brown MW, Daubert JP, et al. Cardiac resynchronization therapy for the prevention of heart failure events. New England Journal of Medicine. 2009;**361**:1329-1338

[13] Abraham WT, Young JB, León AR, Adler S, Bank AJ, Hall SA, et al. Effects of cardiac resynchronization on disease progression in patients with left ventricular systolic dysfunction, an indication for an implantable cardioverter-defibrillator, and mildly

symptomatic chronic heart failure. Circulation. 2004;**110**(18):2864-2868. DOI: 10.1161/01.CIR.0000146336.92331. D1 Epub 2004 Oct 25. PMID: 15505095

[14] Gi-Byoung Nam recent clinical trials on cardiac resynchronization therapy. International Journal of Arrhythmia. 2012;**13**(3):17-21

[15] Normand C, Linde C, Singh J, Dickstein K. Indications for cardiac resynchronization therapy: A comparison of the major international guidelines. JACC: Heart Failure. 2018;**6**:308-316

[16] Stavrakis S, Lazzara R, Thadani U. The benefit of cardiac resynchronization therapy and QRS duration: A meta-analysis. Journal of Cardiovascular Electrophysiology. 2012;**23**:163-168

[17] Kang SH, Oh IY, Kang DY, et al. Cardiac resynchronization therapy and QRS duration: Systematic review, meta-analysis, and meta-regression. Journal of Korean Medical Science. 2015;**30**:24-33

[18] Boriani G, Nesti M, Ziacchi M, Padeletti L. Cardiac resynchronization therapy: An overview on guidelines. Heart Failure Clinics. 2017;**13**:117-137

[19] Chung ES, Leon AR, Tavazzi L, et al. Results of the predictors of response to CRT (PROSPECT) trial. Circulation. 2008;**117**:2608-2616

[20] Prinzen FW, Vernooy K, Auricchio A. Circulation. 2013;**128**(22):2407-2418. DOI: 10.1161/CIRCULATIONAHA. 112.000112

[21] Nakai T, Ikeya Y, Mano H, Kogawa R, Watanabe R, Arai M, et al. Efficacy of cardiac resynchronization therapy in patients with a narrow QRS complex. Journal of Interventional Cardiology. 2021: Article ID 8858836, 7 p. DOI: 10.1155/2021/8858836

[22] Theuns DAMJ, Schaer BA, Caliskan K, Hoeks SE, Sticherling C, Yap SC, et al. Application of the heart failure meta-score to predict prognosis in patients with cardiac resynchronization defibrillators. International Journal of Cardiology. 2021;**330**:73-79. DOI: 10.1016/j.ijcard.2021.01.011

[23] Vernooy K, Cornelussen RNM, Verbeek XAAM, et al. Cardiac resynchronization therapy cures dyssynchronopathy in canine left bundle-branch block hearts. European Heart Journal. 2007;**28**:2148-2155

[24] Cardone-Noott L, Bueno-Orovio A, Minchole A, Zemzemi N, Rodriguez B. Human ventricular activation sequence and the simulation of the electrocardiographic QRS complex and its variability in healthy and intraventricular block conditions. Europace. 2016;**18**:iv4-iv15. DOI: 10.1093/europace/euw346

[25] Ploux S, Eschalier R, Whinnett ZI, et al. Electrical dyssynchrony induced by biventricular pacing: Implications for patient selection and therapy improvement. Heart Rhythm. 2015;**12**: 782-791

[26] Ruschitzka F, Abraham WT, Singh JP, et al. Cardiac resynchronization therapy in heart failure with a narrow QRS complex. The New England Journal of Medicine. 2013;**10**:1395-1405

[27] Thibault B, Harel F, Ducharme A, et al. Cardiac resynchronization therapy in patients with heart failure and a QRS complex <12 msec: The evaluation of resynchronization therapy for heart failure (LESSER-EARTH) trial. Circulation. 2013;**127**:873-881

[28] Van Stipdonk AMW, Horst I, Kloosterman M, et al. QRS area is a strong determinant of outcome in cardiac resynchronization. Circulation. Arrhythmia and Electrophysiology. 2018;**11**:E006497

[29] Van Stipdonk AMW, Vanbelle S, ter Horst IAH, et al. Large variability in

clinical judgement and definitions of left bundle branch block to identify candidates for cardiac resynchronisation therapy. International Journal of Cardiology. 2019;**286**:61-65

[30] Zareba W, Klein H, Cygankiewicz I, et al. Effectiveness of cardiac resynchronization therapy by QRS morphology in the Multicenter Automatic Defibrillator Implantation Trial-Cardiac Resynchronization Therapy (MADIT-CRT). Circulation. 2011;**123**:1061-1072

[31] Gold MR, Thébault C, Linde C, et al. Effect of QRS duration and morphology on cardiac resynchronization therapy outcomes in mild heart failure: Results from the Resynchronization Reverses Remodeling in Systolic Left Ventricular Dysfunction (REVERSE) study. Circulation. 2012;**126**:822-829

[32] Cleland JG, Abraham WT, Linde C, et al. An individual patient meta-analysis of five randomized trials assessing the effects of cardiac resynchronization therapy on morbidity and mortality in patients with symptomatic heart failure. European Heart Journal. 2013;**34**: 3547-3556

[33] Ploux S, Lumens J, Whinnett Z, et al. Noninvasive electrocardiographic mapping to improve patient selection for cardiac resynchronization therapy: Beyond QRS duration and left bundle branch block morphology. Journal of the American College of Cardiology. 2013;**61**:2435-2443

[34] Fantoni C, Kawabata M, Massaro R, et al. Right and left ventricular activation sequence in patients with heart failure and right bundle branch block: A detailed analysis using three-dimensional nonfluoroscopic electroanatomic mapping system. Journal of Cardiovascular Electrophysiology. 2005;**16**:112-119; discussion 120-1

[35] Derval N, Duchateau J, Mahida S, et al. Distinctive left ventricular activations associated with ECG pattern in heart failure patients. Circulation. Arrhythmia and Electrophysiology. 2017;**10**:E005073

[36] Eschalier R, Ploux S, Ritter P, Haissaguerre M, Ellenbogen KA, Bordachar P. Nonspecific intraventricular conduction delay: Definitions, prognosis, and implications for cardiac resynchronization therapy. Heart Rhythm. 2015;**12**:1071-1079

[37] Van Stipdonk A, Mafi Rad M, Luermans JGLM, Crijns HJ, Prinzen FW, Vernooy K. Identifying delayed left ventricular lateral wall activation in patients with non-specific intraventricular conduction delay using coronary venous electroanatomical mapping. Netherlands Heart Journal. 2016;**24**:58-65

[38] Kawata H, Bao H, Curtis JP, et al. Cardiac resynchronization defibrillator therapy for nonspecific intraventricular conduction delay versus right bundle branch block. Journal of the American College of Cardiology. 2019;**73**: 3082-3099

[39] Auricchio A, Lumens J, Prinzen FW. Does cardiac resynchronization therapy benefit patients with right bundle branch block: Cardiac resynchronization therapy has a role in patients with right bundle branch block. Circulation. Arrhythmia and Electrophysiology. 2014;**7**:532-542

[40] Byrne MJ, Helm RH, Daya S, et al. Diminished left ventricular dyssynchrony and impact of resynchronization in failing hearts with right versus left bundle branch block. Journal of the American College of Cardiology. 2007;**50**:1484-1490

[41] Rosenbaum MB. Types of left bundle branch block and their clinical significance. Journal of Electrocardiology. 1969;**2**:197-206

[42] Tzogias L, Steinberg LA, Williams AJ, et al. Electrocardiographic

features and prevalence of bilateral bundle-branch delay. Circulation. Arrhythmia and Electrophysiology. 2014;**7**:640-644

[43] Leeters IPM, Davis A, Zusterzeel R, et al. Left ventricular regional contraction abnormalities by echocardiographic speckle tracking in combined right bundle branch with left anterior fascicular block compared to left bundle branch block. Journal of Electrocardiology. 2016;**49**:353-361

[44] Salden FCWM, Kutyifa V, Stockburger M, Prinzen FW, Vernooy K. Atrioventricular dromotropathy: Evidence for a distinctive entity in heart failure with prolonged PR interval? Europace. 2017;**20**:1067-1077

[45] Kwok CS, Rashid M, Beynon R, et al. Prolonged PR interval, first-degree heart block and adverse cardiovascular outcomes: A systematic review and meta-analysis. Heart. 2016;**102**:672-680

[46] Friedman DJ, Bao H, Spatz ES, Curtis JP, Daubert JP, Al-Khatib SM. Association between a prolonged PR interval and outcomes of cardiac resynchronization therapy: A report from the National Cardiovascular Data Registry. Circulation. 2016;**134**:1617-1628

[47] Januszkiewicz Ł, Vegh E, Borgquist R, et al. Prognostic implication of baseline PR interval in cardiac resynchronization therapy recipients. Heart Rhythm. 2015;**12**:2256-2262

[48] Kutyifa V, Stockburger M, Daubert JP, et al. PR interval identifies clinical response in patients with non-left bundle branch block: A Multicenter Automatic Defibrillator Implantation Trial-Cardiac Resynchronization Therapy substudy. Circulation. Arrhythmia and Electrophysiology. 2014;7:645-651

[49] Lin J, Buhr KA, Kipp R. Effect of PR interval on outcomes following cardiac resynchronization therapy: A secondary analysis of the COMPANION trial. Journal of Cardiovascular Electrophysiology. 2017;**28**:185-191

[50] Olshansky B, Day JD, Sullivan RM, Young P, Galle E, Steinberg JS. Does cardiac resynchronization therapy provide unrecognized benefit in patients with prolonged PR intervals? The impact of restoring atrioventricular synchrony: An analysis from the COMPANION trial. Heart Rhythm. 2012;**9**:34-39

[51] Packer M. Proposal for a new clinical end point to evaluate the efficacy of drugs and devices in the treatment of chronic heart failure. Journal of Cardiac Failure. 2001;**7**:176-182

[52] Jackson T, Claridge S, Behar J, Sammut E, Webb J, Carr-White G, et al. Narrow QRS systolic heart failure: Is there a target for cardiac resynchronization? Expert Review of Cardiovascular Therapy. 2015;**13**(7):783-797. DOI: 10.1586/14779072.2015.1049945

[53] Leenders GE, De Boeck BWL, Teske AJ, et al. Septal rebound stretch is a strong predictor of outcome after cardiac resynchronization therapy. Journal of Cardiac Failure. 2012;**18**:404-412

[54] Gorcsan J III, Anderson CP, Tayal B, et al. Systolic stretch characterizes the electromechanical substrate responsive to cardiac resynchronization therapy. JACC. Cardiovascular Imaging. 2019;**12**:1741-1752

[55] Beela AS, Serkan U, Ciarka A, et al. Assessment of mechanical dyssynchrony can improve the prognostic value of guideline based patient selection for cardiac resynchronization therapy. European Heart Journal Cardiovascular Imaging. 2019;**20**:66-74

[56] Tracy CM, Epstein AE, Darbar D, et al. 2012 ACCF/AHA/HRS focused update incorporated into the ACCF/AHA/HRS 2008 guidelines for device

based therapy of cardiac rhythm abnormalities: A report of the American College of Cardiology Foundation/ American Heart Association Task Force on Practice Guidelines and the Heart Rhythm Society. Journal of the American College of Cardiology. 2013;**61**:e6-e75

[57] Ponikowski P, Voors AA, Anker SD, et al. 2016 ESC guidelines for the diagnosis and treatment of acute and chronic heart failure: The Task Force for the Diagnosis and Treatment of Acute and Chronic Heart Failure of the European Society of Cardiology (ESC): Developed with the special contribution of the Heart Failure Association (HFA) of the ESC. European Heart Journal. 2016;**37**:2129-2200

[58] De Boeck BWL, Teske AJ, Meine M, Leenders GE, Cramer MJ, Prinzen FW, et al. Septal rebound stretch reflects the functional substrate to cardiac resynchronization therapy and predicts volumetric and neurohormonal response. European Journal of Heart Failure. 2009;**11**:863-871

[59] Lumens J, Tayal B, Walmsley J, Delgado-Montero A, Huntjens PR, Schwartzman D, et al. Differentiating electromechanical from non-electrical substrates of mechanical discoordination to identify responders to cardiac resynchronization therapy. Circulation. Cardiovascular Imaging. 2015;**8**:e003744

[60] Risum N, Tayal B, Hansen TF, Bruun NE, Jensen MT, Lauridsen TK, et al. Identification of typical left bundle branch block contraction by strain echocardiography is additive to electrocardiography in prediction of long-term outcome after cardiac resynchronization therapy. Journal of the American College of Cardiology. 2015;**66**:631-641

[61] Prinzen FW, Hunter WC, Wyman BT, Mcveigh ER. Mapping of regional myocardial strain and work during ventricular pacing: Experimental study using magnetic resonance imaging tagging. Journal of the American College of Cardiology. 1999;**33**:1735-1742

[62] Leenders GE, Lumens J, Cramer MJ, De Boeck BWL, Doevendans PA, Delhaas T, et al. Septal deformation patterns delineate mechanical dyssynchrony and regional differences in contractility analysis of patient data using a computer model. Circulation. Heart Failure. 2012;**5**:87-96

[63] Galli E, Leclercq C, Fournet M, Hubert A, Bernard A, Smiseth OA, et al. Value of myocardial work estimation in the prediction of response to cardiac resynchronization therapy. Journal of the American Society of Echocardiography. 2018;**31**:220-230

[64] Smiseth OA, Russell K, Skulstad H. The role of echocardiography in quantification of left ventricular dyssynchrony: State of the art and future directions Otto. European Heart Journal Cardiovascular Imaging. 2012;**13**:61-68

[65] Salden OAE, Zweerink A, Wouters P, Allaart CP, Geelhoed B, de Lange FJ, et al. The value of septal rebound stretch analysis for the prediction of volumetric response to cardiac resynchronization therapy. European Heart Journal—Cardiovascular Imaging. 2021;**22**(1):37-45. DOI: 10.1093/ehjci/jeaa190

[66] Van Sant J, Horst IAH, Wijers SC, Mast TP, Leenders GE, Doevendans PA, et al. Measurements of electrical and mechanical dyssynchrony are both essential to improve prediction of CRT response. Journal of Electrocardiology. 2015;**48**:601-608

[67] Salden OAE, Vernooy K, van Stipdonk AMW, Cramer MJ, Prinzen FW, Meine M. Strategies to improve selection of patients without typical left bundle branch block for cardiac resynchronization therapy. JACC: Clinical Electrophysiology.

2020;**6**(2):129-142. ISSN 2405-500X. DOI: 10.1016/j.jacep.2019.11.018

[68] Torrent-Guasp F, Kocica MJ, Corno AF, Komeda M, Carreras-Costa F, Flotats A, et al. Towards new understanding of the heart structure and function. European Journal of Cardio-Thoracic Surgery. 2005;**27**:191-201

[69] Greenbaum RA, Ho SY, Gibson DG, Becker AE, Anderson RH. Left ventricular fibre architecture in man. British Heart Journal. 1981;**45**(3):248-263

[70] Yettram A, Vinson CA, Gibson DG. Effect of myocardial fibre architecture on the behaviour of the human left ventricle in diastole. Journal of Biomedical Engineering. 1983;**5**:321-328

[71] Antzelevitch C, Fish J. Electrical heterogeneity within the ventricular wall. Basic Research in Cardiology. 2001;**96**:517-527

[72] Cassidy D, Vassallo J, Miller J, Poll D, Buxton A, Marchinski F, et al. Endocardial catheter mapping in patients in sinus rhythm: Relationship to underlying heart disease and ventricular arrhythmias. Circulation. 1986;**73**: 645-652

[73] Tournoux F, Donal E, Leclercq C, De Place C, Crocq C, Solnon A, et al. Concordance between mechanical and electrical dyssynchrony in heart failure patients: A function of the underlying cardiomyopathy? Journal of Cardiovascular Electrophysiology. 2007;**18**: 1022-1027

[74] Leyva F. Cardiac resynchronization therapy guided by cardiovascular magnetic resonance. Journal of Cardiovascular Magnetic Resonance. 2010;**12**:64. DOI: 10.1186/1532-429X-12-64

[75] Foley PW, Khadjooi K, Ward JA, Smith RE, Stegemann B, Frenneaux MP, et al. Radial dyssynchrony assessed by cardiovascular magnetic resonance in relation to left ventricular function, myocardial scarring and QRS duration in patients with heart failure. Journal of Cardiovascular Magnetic Resonance. 2009;**11**(1):50-56

[76] White JA, Yee R, Yuan X, Krahn A, Skanes A, Parker M, et al. Delayed enhancement magnetic resonance imaging predicts response to cardiac resynchronization therapy in patients with intraventricular dyssynchrony. Journal of the American College of Cardiology. 2006;**48**(10):1953-1960

[77] Chalil S, Foley P, Muyhaldeen S, Patel K, Yousef Z, Smith R, et al. Late gadolinium enhancement-cardiovascular magnetic resonance as a predictor of response to cardiac resynchronization therapy in patients with ischaemic cardiomyopathy. Europace. 2007;**9**: 1031-1037

[78] Pezel T, Mika D, Logeart D, et al. Characterization of non-response to cardiac resynchronization therapy by post-procedural computed tomography. Pacing and Clinical Electrophysiology. 2021;**44**:135-144. DOI: 10.1111/pace.14134

[79] Galand V, Ghoshhajra B, Szymonifka J, Das S, Orencole M, Barré V, et al. Left ventricular wall thickness assessed by cardiac computed tomography and cardiac resynchronization therapy outcomes. EP Europace. 2020;**22**(3):401-411. DOI: 10.1093/europace/euz322

[80] McAlister FA, Ezekowitz J, Hooton N, et al. Cardiac resynchronization therapy for patients with left ventricular systolic dysfunction: A systematic review. JAMA. 2007;**297**: 2502-2514

[81] Fornwalt BK, Sprague WW, BeDell P, et al. Agreement is poor among current criteria used to define response to cardiac resynchronization

therapy. Circulation. 2010;**121**: 1985-1991

[82] Emerek K, Friedman DJ, Sørensen PL, et al. Vectorcardiographic QRS area is associated with long-term outcome after cardiac resynchronization therapy. Heart Rhythm. 2019;**16**:213-219

[83] Engels EB, Végh EM, Van Deursen CJ, Vernooy K, Singh JP, Prinzen FW. T-wave area predicts response to cardiac resynchronization therapy in patients with left bundle branch block. Journal of Cardiovascular Electrophysiology. 2015;**26**:176-183

[84] Van Deursen CJM, Vernooy K, Dudink E, et al. Vectorcardiographic QRS area as a novel predictor of response to cardiac resynchronization therapy. Journal of Electrocardiology. 2015;**48**:45-52

[85] Maass AH, Vernooy K, Wijers SC, et al. Refining success of cardiac resynchronization therapy using a simple score predicting the amount of reverse ventricular remodelling: Results from the Markers and Response to CRT (MARC) study. Ep Europace. 2018;**20**: e1-e10

[86] Pfeiffer ER, Tangney JR, Omens JH, McCulloch AD. Biomechanics of cardiac electromechanical coupling and mechanoelectric feedback. Journal of Biomechanical Engineering. 2014; **136**(2):021007. DOI: 10.1115/1.4026221

[87] Torrent-Guasp F. Anatomía Funcional del Corazón. Madrid: PazMontalbo; 1957

[88] Torrent-Guasp F. An Experimental Approach in Heart Dynamics Physiology and Pharmacology. Eugene Talmadge Hospital. Augusta (GA). Madrid: S. Aguirre Torre; 1959

[89] Streeter DD, Torrent-Guasp F. Geodesic paths in the left ventricle of the mammalian heart. Circulation. 1973;**48**:471-477

[90] Streeter DD, Powers WE, Ross MA, Torrent-Guasp F. Three-dimensional fiber orientation in the mammalian left ventricular wall. In: Barn J, Noordegraf A, Raines J, editors. Cardiovascular System Dynamics. Cambridge: MIT Press; 1978. p. 73

[91] Torrent-Guasp F. Estructura y función del corazón. Revista Española de Cardiología. 1998;**51**:91-102

[92] Ballester-Rodés M, Flotats A, Torrent-Guasp F, Carrió-Gasset I, Ballester-Alomar M, Carreras F, et al. The sequence of regional ventricular motion. European Journal of Cardio-Thoracic Surgery. 2006;29(Suppl_1):S139–S144. DOI: 10.1016/j.ejcts.2006.02.058

[93] Sengupta PP, Khandheria BK, Narula J. Twist and untwist mechanics of the left ventricle. Heart Failure Clinics. 2008;**4**(3):315-324. DOI: 10.1016/j.hfc.2008.03.001

[94] Reddy VY, Miller MA, Neuzil P, et al. Cardiac resynchronization therapy with wireless left ventricular endocardial pacing: The SELECT-LV study. Journal of the American College of Cardiology. 2017;**69**:2119-2129

[95] Shetty AK, Sohal M, Chen Z, et al. A comparison of left ventricular endocardial, multisite, and multipolar epicardial cardiac resynchronization: An acute haemodynamic and electro-anatomical study. Europace. 2014;**16**: 873-879

[96] Morgan JM, Biffi M, Gellér L, et al. ALternate Site Cardiac ResYNChronization (ALSYNC): A prospective and multicentre study of left ventricular endocardial pacing for cardiac resynchronization therapy. European Heart Journal. 2016;**37**: 2118-2127

[97] Auricchio A, Delnoy PP, Butter C, et al. Feasibility, safety, and short-term outcome of leadless ultrasoundbased

endocardial left ventricular resynchronization in heart failure patients: Results of the wireless stimulation endocardially for CRT (WiSE-CRT) study. Europace. 2014;**16**:681-688

[98] Narula OS. Longitudinal dissociation in the Hisbundle. Bundle branch block due to asynchronousconduction within the His bundle in man. Circulation. 1977;**56**:996-1006

[99] Lustgarten DL, Calame S, Crespo EM, Calame J, Lobel R, Spector PS. Electrical resynchronization induced by direct His-bundle pacing. Heart Rhythm. 2010;**7**:15-21

[100] Deshmukh P, Casavant DA, Romanyshyn M, Anderson K. Permanent, direct His-bundle pacing: A novel approach to cardiac pacing in patients with normal His-Purkinje activation. Circulation. 2000;**101**:869-877

[101] Barba-Pichardo R, Manovel Sanchez A, Fernandez-Gomez JM, Morina-Vazquez P, Venegas-Gamero J, Herrera-Carranza M. Ventricular resynchronization therapy by direct His-bundle pacing using an internal cardioverter defibrillator. Europace. 2013;**15**:83-88

[102] Sharma PS, Naperkowski A, Oren JW, Storm RH, Ellenbogen KA, Vijayaraman P. Permanent His-bundle pacing is feasible, safe, and superior to right ventricular pacing in routine clinical practice. Heart Rhythm. 2014;**0**:1-8

[103] Lee MY, Yeshwant SC, Lustgarten DL. Honing in on optimal ventricular pacing sites: An argument for his bundle pacing. Current Treatment Options in Cardiovascular Medicine. 2015;**17**:372

[104] Upadhyay GA, Cherian T, Shatz DY, et al. Intracardiac delineation of septal conduction in left bundle-branch block patterns. Circulation. 2019;**139**:1876-1888

[105] Teng AE, Massoud L, Ajijola OA. Physiological mechanisms of QRS narrowing in bundle branch block patients undergoing permanent His bundle pacing. Journal of Electrocardiology. 2016;**49**:644-648

[106] Arnold AD, Shun-Shin MJ, Keene D, et al. His resynchronization versus biventricular pacing inpatients with heart failure and left bundle branchblock. Journal of the American College of Cardiology. 2018;**72**:3112-3122

[107] Vijayaraman P, Herweg B, Ellenbogen KA, Gajek J. His-optimized cardiac resynchronizationtherapy to maximize electrical resynchronization: a feasibility study. Circulation: Arrhythmia Electrophysiology. 2019;**12**:e006934

Chapter 6

High-Power, Short-Duration Ablation in the Treatment of Atrial Fibrillation Patients

Nándor Szegedi and László Gellér

Abstract

Catheter ablation is the cornerstone of the rhythm control treatment of atrial fibrillation (AF). During this procedure, creating a contiguous and durable lesion set is essential to achieve good long-term results. Radiofrequency lesions are created in two phases: resistive and conductive heating. The ablation catheters and the generators have undergone impressive technical developments to enable homogenous and good-quality lesion creation. Despite recent years' achievements, the durable isolation of the pulmonary veins remains a challenge. These days, intensive research aims to evaluate the role of high-power radiofrequency applications in the treatment of patients with cardiac arrhythmias. The use of high-power, short-duration applications might result in a uniform, transmural lesion set. It is associated with shorter procedure time, shorter left atrial, and fluoroscopy time than low-power ablation. This technique was also associated with a better clinical outcome, possibly due to the better durability of lesions. Multiple clinical studies have proven the safety and efficacy of high-power, short-duration PVI.

Keywords: catheter ablation, high power, short duration, lesion formation, atrial fibrillation

1. Introduction

Atrial fibrillation (AF) is the most common sustained cardiac arrhythmia. AF is associated with a higher risk of mortality, and it is one of the major causes of stroke, heart failure, sudden death, and cardiovascular morbidity worldwide [1, 2]. Thus, appropriate management of this arrhythmia and underlying diseases is essential.

Catheter ablation is the cornerstone of the rhythm control treatment of AF by isolating the pulmonary veins from the left atrium (pulmonary vein isolation; PVI). During this procedure, creating a contiguous and durable lesion set is essential to achieve good long-term results [3, 4]. When applying radiofrequency (RF) ablations, the lesions are created in two phases: resistive and conductive heating of the myocardial tissue [5]. Both the ablation catheters and the generators have undergone impressive technical developments to reach homogenous and good-quality lesion creation. Despite recent years' technological developments, the durable isolation of the pulmonary veins remains a challenge. Moreover, procedural complications also remained a significant issue [6–8].

Nowadays, the use of high-power (HP) radiofrequency applications is in the center of scientific research. High-power, short-duration (HPSD) ablation might result in a more uniform, transmural lesion set [9]. Thus, it can reduce procedure time and seems to be non-inferior compared to low-power (LP) ablation. This technique was associated with a better clinical outcome, possibly due to the better durability of PVI [10]. Multiple clinical studies have proven the safety and efficacy of high-power, short-duration PVI for AF ablation.

In this chapter, we will introduce the theoretical background of HPSD ablation, and we also aim to discuss the main differences with low-power ablations, also mentioning some relevant clinical trials.

2. Theoretical background of radiofrequency lesion formation

Radiofrequency catheter ablation is the first-line treatment choice for most symptomatic arrhythmias. The tissue injury caused by this energy source is thermally mediated, resulting in discrete and homogeneous lesions.

2.1 Radiofrequency energy delivery and tissue heating

The standard RF generator used for catheter ablation produces a sine wave alternating current at 350–500 kHz. The RF energy delivery is usually unipolar between the ablation catheter's tip electrode and a large surface indifferent electrode applied to the patient's skin. During RF energy delivery, the alternating electrical current traverses from the ablation catheter's tip electrode through the intervening tissue to the indifferent electrode. The passage of the electric current through the tissue results in electromagnetic heating, termed resistive heating. Resistive heating is proportional to the square of the current density; current density is inversely proportional to the square of the distance from the ablation electrode. Therefore, power dissipation per unit volume decreases dramatically with the distance, and resistive heating decreases with the distance from the ablation electrode to the fourth power. Since the region of the highest current density is at the tissue below the ablation electrode, resistive heating of the tissue only occurs in a thin layer within a very close vicinity to the ablation electrode. Deeper tissue heating occurs as a result of passive heat conduction from this narrow resistive heating zone, termed conductive heating (**Figure 1**). Temperatures above 50°C are required for irreversible myocardial injury. Of note, a non-negligible part of the delivered energy will be lost as a consequence of convective heat loss to the blood pool surrounding the ablation electrode [5].

2.2 Factors influencing radiofrequency lesion creation

Lesion formation is dependent on optimal electrode-tissue contact force (CF), RF power, size of ablation catheter tip electrode, and the duration of RF delivery.

The role of the ablation catheter tip size will not be discussed in this chapter, as the vast majority of the electrophysiology laboratories only use 3.5–4-mm tip electrodes in everyday practice, and large-tip electrodes are utilized less commonly.

Lesion size is directly proportional to the electrode-tissue contact temperature. Therefore, those factors that increase the temperature at the electrode-tissue interface (e.g., RF power and contact force) will also increase the lesion size.

It is known that the lesion size is proportional to RF power, as a higher RF power results in a larger current density at the ablation electrode leading to greater tissue heating. However, the deliverable power (and time) might be limited by an impedance rise that occurs when the temperature at the electrode-tissue interface reaches 100°C. This impedance rise can be prevented by maintaining the electrode-tissue

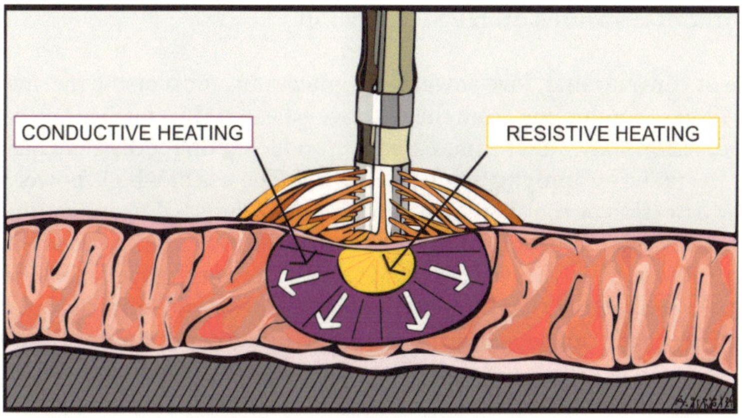

Figure 1.
Phases of lesion formation during radiofrequency ablation. The first phase is the resistive heating occurring in a thin layer of the tissue contacting the ablation electrode. The second phase is the heat conduction from the resistively heated zone to the more distant tissue layers (conductive heating).

interface temperature below 100°C by cooling the tip of the ablation catheter. A landmark *in vivo* study was presented by Nakagawa et al. [11]. They evaluated the role of presence or absence of catheter tip irrigation in eleven anesthetized dogs' tight muscles. They executed temperature measurements on the catheter-tissue surface and tissue temperatures in 3.5 mm and 7 mm depth. The main findings were that in the case of applications with irrigation of the catheter tip, electrode and electrode-tissue interface temperatures were consistently lower than the tissue temperature at 3.5 mm depth. Moreover, lesion sizes were larger in the case of irrigated ablations, most likely because they could deliver higher-power applications in this group [11, 12].

Later, studies concluded that irrigation minimally affects lesion size by cooling the tissue surface (when the applied power is the same). Larger lesions may only be created with the use of irrigation by making the delivery of higher-power levels possible. This is especially important in case of low blood flow areas where high temperatures are reached at relatively low-power levels, resulting in insufficient lesion formation. In such areas, irrigation decreases temperature during ablation and therefore makes the delivery of a higher power possible [13].

When tissue contact is poor, a larger surface area of the ablation electrode is exposed to the circulating blood pool, which results in less-efficient tissue heating. Conversely, good tissue contact results in a larger area where catheter touches the tissue and less amount of current will be lost to the blood pool. In case of low CF, a higher power might be necessary to reach an optimal degree of tissue heating. On the other hand, similarly, good lesion formation can be produced even with smaller CF in case of high-power applications [5]. A few years ago, contact force-sensing ablation catheters were introduced and nowadays, their use is a part of everyday practice. They allow to reach better durability of lesions and thus facilitate the procedure in terms of achieving better safety and efficacy [3, 14–16].

Finally, an essential determinant of lesion size is the duration of RF application. The rate of tissue heating at the electrode-tissue contact point is rapid, and steady-state temperatures are reached within a few seconds in the resistive heating zone. Conversely, deeper tissue sites have a much slower rate of temperature rise due to the time required for conductive heating. Thus, the lesion growth is rapid in the first few seconds but much slower thereafter. Studies have demonstrated that the half-time of lesion growth is approximately 7–10 s, and maximum lesion size is achieved after 30–40 s of RF energy delivery [5].

3. Experimental studies on HPSD ablation

In case of conventional, low-power RF applications, most of the thermal injury is a result of heat conduction from the resistively heated thin surface layer. On the other hand, lesion size could be increased by producing direct resistive heating deeper in the tissue by applying higher RF power. The use of a high-power level is allowed by irrigation of the ablation electrode with saline. Saline irrigation maintains a low electrode-tissue interface temperature during radiofrequency application at high power, which prevents a rapid temperature and impedance rise.

Nakagawa et al. found that by applying higher power with an irrigated catheter, a higher temperature can be measured at 3.5 mm tissue depth than at the electrode-tissue interface, which indicates that direct resistive heating occurred deeper in the tissue (rather than by conduction of heat from the surface) [11]. Other early studies also found that high-power ablations are effective; however, there was a concern regarding the safety of the procedures based on the animal study results [17]. This seems justified since high-power ablations necessitate reliable real-time feedback on lesion formation to avoid serious complications. Lesion-predicting parameters were not available before the contact force era; therefore, research interest regarding high-power RF ablation decreased transiently. However, after introducing CF-sensing catheters and lesion-predicting parameters, the topic became interesting again. If high power is applied for a long duration, it leads to a big resistive heating zone to which a large conductive heating zone is added, resulting in the creation of extensive lesions. Therefore, high-power ablations should only be applied for a short time to avoid the injury of extracardiac structures.

Nowadays, intensive research is going on examining high-power, short-duration RF ablation technology. Bourier et al. [9] showed that HPSD ablation results in a different lesion geometry (e.g., larger diameters but smaller depth) compared to conventional lower-power ablation. Still, the depth of the high-power applications seems sufficient to reach transmural lesions in the atria (**Figure 2**). Moreover, the larger diameters might improve the chance of creating a contiguous lesion set [9].

Two other preclinical studies evaluated the efficacy and safety of very high-power, short-duration RF ablation (90-W power applied for 4 s) compared to low-power, long-duration ablation in swine models. Both studies showed that HPSD ablation results in improved lesion continuity, lesion transmurality, and shorter ablation time, while the safety profile is comparable to conventional low-power ablation [10, 18].

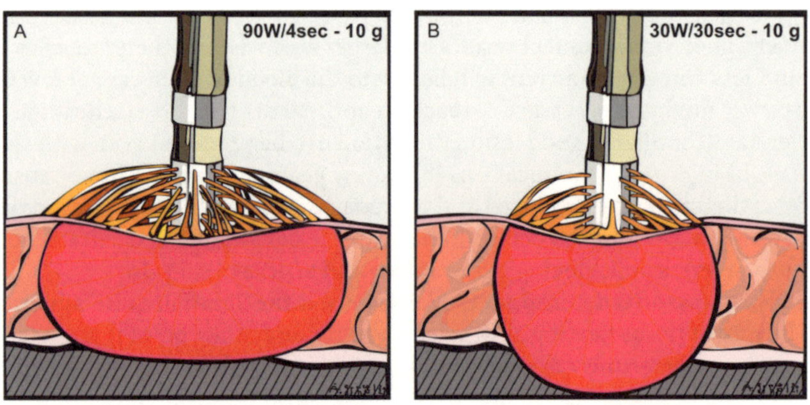

Figure 2.
Properties of lesions created by high-power, short-duration and low-power, long-duration radiofrequency ablation. The high-power, short-duration ablation (panel A) results in a different lesion geometry (e.g., larger diameters but smaller depth) compared to conventional lower-power ablation (panel B). Still, the depth of the high-power application's lesion seems sufficient to reach transmurality in the atria.

4. Clinical trials evaluating HPSD PVI

4.1 Ablation index-guided PVI with HPSD applications

According to previous studies, ablation index (AI) is a valuable marker of lesion creation during PVI procedure, minimizing the risk of AF recurrence after ablation [14, 19]. AI is calculated by a weighted formula including CF, RF time, and power so that a higher-power application can reach target AI with a shorter duration and even with high energy, RF applications' lesion creation can be monitored in real time properly. Of note, the AI is validated up to 45 W; thus, lesion creation can be reliably monitored with AI at a maximal power of 45 W. The decrease of RF time per application theoretically makes the maintenance of a stable catheter position at the given site easier, resulting in a better lesion quality. It is well known that HPSD ablation results in a different lesion geometry (e.g., larger diameters but smaller depth) compared to conventional lower-power ablation. Still, the depth of the HP applications is sufficient to reach transmural lesions in the atria. The power used for ablation can be varied based on the operating physician's decision. As we will show in this subchapter, 45–50 W was used in the majority of trials.

The use of high-power (HP) RF applications can reduce procedural time and seemed to be non-inferior to low-power (LP) ablation in a multicenter study [20]. Vassallo et al. investigated patients who underwent AF ablation with HP (50 W on the anterior wall and 45 W elsewhere in the left atrium) or LP (30 W) RF ablation power settings. HPSD was safe and efficient compared with LP ablation and was associated with a reduced procedural time and total RF time. They also concluded that HPSD might reduce the chance of esophageal injury and it may also reduce the recurrence of atrial tachyarrythmias [21]. The PVI procedure time was also decreased significantly with HP (50 W) ablation compared to conventional LP (30 W) ablation settings in a study published by Bunch et al. [22].

We would like to highlight a prospective randomized trial conducted by Wielandts et al. [23]. They randomized 96 AF patients to HPSD (45 W) or LPLD (35 W), CLOSE protocol-guided PVI and found that fluoroscopy dose and RF time are lower in case of HPSD ablation. There was no difference in terms of six-month AF-free survival between the two groups. On the other hand, postprocedural endoscopic evaluation of esophageal lesions drew attention to a narrower safety margin at the posterior wall using high power, especially when applying higher CF and reaching higher AI values [23].

Finally, we would like to mention a recent meta-analysis of 15 studies evaluating PVI with HPSD *versus* LP ablation technique. Overall, data of 3718 patients were included in the analysis. The main result is that freedom from atrial arrhythmias was higher in case of HPSD RF ablation when compared with conventional LP RF ablation. Acute PV reconnection was lower and first-pass isolation was higher with HPSD. There was no statistically significant difference in total complications between the two groups. Total procedure duration, fluoroscopy duration, and RF ablation time were all significantly lower in HPSD ablation [24].

4.2 HPSD safety endpoints: esophageal lesions

Esophageal lesions are not rare after RF point-by-point PVI, even with the use of CF sensing catheters [25, 26]. A rare but potentially lethal complication of pulmonary vein isolation is atrio-esophageal fistula [6]. Thus, besides improving efficacy, reducing the possibility of causing esophageal lesions should be the main goal of technological developments. High-power RF applications have a larger resistive heating zone, but conductive heating does not significantly affect the lesion creation if the application is kept short. On the other hand, one has to keep in mind that applying high power for a longer duration can cause extensive tissue injury damaging peri-cardiac structures such as the lung or the esophagus.

A study involving 85 patients who underwent PVI with 35-W power using CF-sensing catheters and AI guidance showed that the occurrence of esophageal injury after PVI is markedly low (1.2%), even in those cases where an intraesophageal temperature rise was detected during the procedure. They concluded that their strategy of delivering contiguous, relatively high-power, and short-duration radiofrequency applications is safe even at the posterior wall [27]. Two other larger trials involving 355 and 271 patients who underwent AI-guided PVI with 45–50-W power also concluded that HPSD technique is relatively safe. Esophageal lesions had a similar incidence in HPSD group as in the low-power group, and there was a low incidence of esophageal temperature elevation in the HPSD group [28]. They concluded that HPSD might even have a protective effect avoiding incidental esophageal injury due to the smaller lesion depth [29]. Of note, this is only true if high-power applications are kept very short on the posterior wall, but longer-duration ablations might lead to severe complications.

5. Very high-power, short-duration ablation of AF

The impressive safety and efficacy profile of high-power, short-duration PVI procedures performed with 45–50 W formed a claim to even higher-power ablations with the potential promise of making procedures even shorter while maintaining safety and efficacy. For sure, ablations with very high power should be carried out with caution to avoid the use of high CF values. Appropriate irrigation is also essential to use this technology, which is solved at the recent version of the CoolFlow (Biosense Webster) pump used for 90-W ablations with the QDOT Micro (Biosense Webster) catheter. Because of the very short time of the applications, lesion-predicting parameters such as AI do not work for this type of ablation. Visual tags of the ablated area are located at the spot where the application was started (**Figure 3**).

Long-term results of such clinical trials are likely to be published in the near future. Here, we would like to mention two studies dealing with very high-power, short-duration PVI.

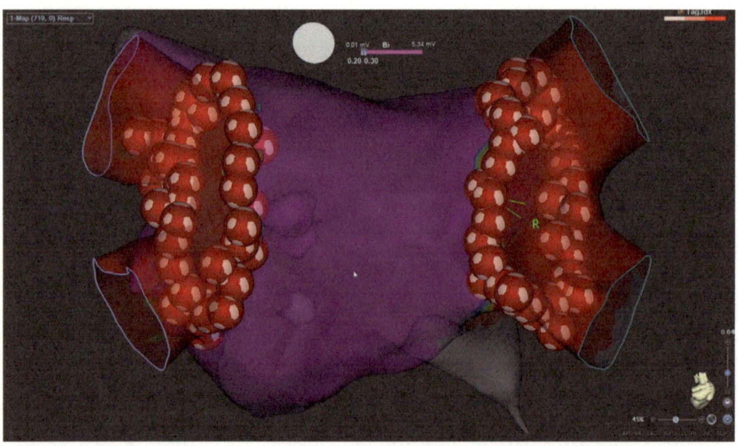

Figure 3.
Electroanatomical map of a successful pulmonary vein isolation performed with very high-power, short-duration ablation technique. All ablation tags represent single applications with 90-W power for 4 s.

Kottmaier et al. [30] compared PVI procedures performed with 70 W *versus* 30–40 W. Very high-power applications were terminated at 5 and 7 s on the posterior and anterior walls, respectively. HPSD ablation demonstrated a comparable safety profile to conventional ablation. Moreover, HPSD ablation led to significantly fewer arrhythmia recurrences after the one-year, follow-up period. Of course, RF time and procedural time were also significantly shortened by the use of HPSD [30].

A prospective, multicenter, single-arm study was published by Reddy et al. [31], aiming to evaluate the safety and efficacy of very HPSD pulmonary vein isolation with 90 W. All applications were terminated after 4 s. They demonstrated the clinical feasibility and safety of very high-power, short-duration ablation, with very low procedure and fluoroscopy times [31].

6. Conclusions

Pulmonary vein isolation is the cornerstone of rhythm-control therapy for atrial fibrillation. A few years ago, new technologies such as contact force-sensing ablation catheters were introduced and became a part of everyday practice. The routine use of CF-sensing ablation catheters improved the arrhythmia-free survival after PVI. However, the recurrence rate of atrial tachyarrhythmias remained a substantial issue. The durability of PVI depends on the accurate lesion creation and contiguity of lesions. The use of high-power, short-duration radiofrequency applications might enable the operators to create a more uniform, more contiguous lesion set; therefore, a more durable PVI can be achieved. This high rate of durable PV isolation is expected to be associated with improved clinical outcomes for atrial fibrillation ablation. Clinical studies uniformly showed that PVI with high-power, short-duration technique is safe and effective and is associated with shorter procedure and ablation times when compared with conventional low-power RF ablation. The long-term efficacy of very HPSD ablation is not available at the moment and needs to be confirmed by further trials.

Acknowledgements

Project no. NVKP_16-1–2016-0017 ('National Heart Program') has been implemented with the support provided by the National Research, Development, and Innovation Fund of Hungary, financed under the NVKP_16 funding scheme. The research was financed by the Thematic Excellence Programme (2020-4.1.1.-TKP2020) of the Ministry for Innovation and Technology in Hungary, within the framework of the Therapeutic Development and Bioimaging thematic programmes of the Semmelweis University.

Conflict of interest

The authors declare no conflict of interest.

Author details

Nándor Szegedi* and László Gellér
Heart and Vascular Center, Semmelweis University, Budapest, Hungary

*Address all correspondence to: nandorszegedi@gmail.com

References

[1] Hindricks G, Potpara T, Dagres N, Arbelo E, Bax JJ, Blomstrom-Lundqvist C, et al. 2020 ESC guidelines for the diagnosis and management of atrial fibrillation developed in collaboration with the European Association for Cardio-Thoracic Surgery (EACTS). European Heart Journal. 2021;**42**(5):373-498

[2] Benjamin EJ, Wolf PA, D'Agostino RB, Silbershatz H, Kannel WB, Levy D. Impact of atrial fibrillation on the risk of death: The Framingham Heart Study. Circulation. 1998;**98**(10):946-952

[3] Szegedi N, Gellér L. New results in catheter ablation for atrial fibrillation. In: Cismaru G, editor. Epidemiology and Treatment of Atrial Fibrillation. Rijeka: IntechOpen; 2019

[4] Das M, Loveday JJ, Wynn GJ, Gomes S, Saeed Y, Bonnett LJ, et al. Ablation index, a novel marker of ablation lesion quality: prediction of pulmonary vein reconnection at repeat electrophysiology study and regional differences in target values. Europace. 2017;**19**(5):775-783

[5] Nath S, DiMarco JP, Haines DE. Basic aspects of radiofrequency catheter ablation. Journal of Cardiovascular Electrophysiology. 1994;**5**(10):863-876

[6] Szegedi N, Suhai IF, Perge P, Sallo Z, Hartyanszky I, Merkely B, et al. Atrio-esophageal fistula clinically presented as pericardial-esophageal fistula. Journal of Interventional Cardiac Electrophysiology. 2021;**61**(3):623-624

[7] Szegedi N, Szeplaki G, Herczeg S, Tahin T, Sallo Z, Nagy VK, et al. Repeat procedure is a new independent predictor of complications of atrial fibrillation ablation. Europace. 2019;**21**(5):732-737

[8] Casado-Arroyo R, Chierchia GB, Conte G, Levinstein M, Sieira J, Rodriguez-Manero M, et al. Phrenic nerve paralysis during cryoballoon ablation for atrial fibrillation: A comparison between the first- and second-generation balloon. Heart Rhythm. 2013;**10**(9):1318-1324

[9] Bourier F, Duchateau J, Vlachos K, Lam A, Martin CA, Takigawa M, et al. High-power short-duration versus standard radiofrequency ablation: Insights on lesion metrics. Journal of Cardiovascular Electrophysiology. 2018;**29**(11):1570-1575

[10] Barkagan M, Contreras-Valdes FM, Leshem E, Buxton AE, Nakagawa H, Anter E. High-power and short-duration ablation for pulmonary vein isolation: Safety, efficacy, and long-term durability. Journal of Cardiovascular Electrophysiology. 2018;**29**(9):1287-1296

[11] Nakagawa H, Yamanashi WS, Pitha JV, Arruda M, Wang X, Ohtomo K, et al. Comparison of in vivo tissue temperature profile and lesion geometry for radiofrequency ablation with a saline-irrigated electrode versus temperature control in a canine thigh muscle preparation. Circulation. 1995;**91**(8):2264-2273

[12] Kongsgaard E, Steen T, Jensen O, Aass H, Amlie JP. Temperature guided radiofrequency catheter ablation of myocardium: Comparison of catheter tip and tissue temperatures in vitro. Pacing and Clinical Electrophysiology. 1997;**20**(5 Pt 1):1252-1260

[13] Wittkampf FH, Nakagawa H. RF catheter ablation: Lessons on lesions. Pacing and Clinical Electrophysiology. 2006;**29**(11):1285-1297

[14] Taghji P, El Haddad M, Phlips T, Wolf M, Knecht S, Vandekerckhove Y, et al. Evaluation of a strategy aiming to enclose the pulmonary veins with

contiguous and optimized radiofrequency lesions in paroxysmal atrial fibrillation: A pilot study. JACC: Clinical Electrophysiology. 2018;**4**(1):99-108

[15] Nakagawa H, Jackman WM. The role of contact force in atrial fibrillation ablation. Journal of Atrial Fibrillation. 2014;**7**(1):1027

[16] Ikeda A, Nakagawa H, Lambert H, Shah DC, Fonck E, Yulzari A, et al. Relationship between catheter contact force and radiofrequency lesion size and incidence of steam pop in the beating canine heart: electrogram amplitude, impedance, and electrode temperature are poor predictors of electrode-tissue contact force and lesion size. Circulation. Arrhythmia and Electrophysiology. 2014;**7**(6):1174-1180

[17] Peng J, Madrid AH, Palmeiro A, Rebollo JM, Limon L, Nannini S, et al. Saline irrigated catheter ablation for pulmonary vein isolation in pigs: an experimental model. Pacing and Clinical Electrophysiology. 2004;**27**(4):495-501

[18] Leshem E, Zilberman I, Tschabrunn CM, Barkagan M, Contreras-Valdes FM, Govari A, et al. High-power and short-duration ablation for pulmonary vein isolation: Biophysical characterization. JACC: Clinical Electrophysiology. 2018;**4**(4):467-479

[19] Hussein A, Das M, Riva S, Morgan M, Ronayne C, Sahni A, et al. Use of ablation index-guided ablation results in high rates of durable pulmonary vein isolation and freedom from arrhythmia in persistent atrial fibrillation patients. Circulation. Arrhythmia and Electrophysiology. 2018;**11**(9):e006576

[20] Dhillon G, Ahsan S, Honarbakhsh S, Lim W, Baca M, Graham A, et al. A multicentered evaluation of ablation at higher power guided by ablation index: Establishing ablation targets for pulmonary vein isolation. Journal of Cardiovascular Electrophysiology. 2019;**30**(3):357-365

[21] Vassallo F, Cunha C, Serpa E, Meigre LL, Carloni H, Simoes A Jr, et al. Comparison of high-power short-duration (HPSD) ablation of atrial fibrillation using a contact force-sensing catheter and conventional technique: Initial results. Journal of Cardiovascular Electrophysiology. 2019;**30**(10): 1877-1883

[22] Bunch TJ, May HT, Bair TL, Crandall BG, Cutler MJ, Mallender C, et al. Long-term outcomes after low power, slower movement versus high power, faster movement irrigated-tip catheter ablation for atrial fibrillation. Heart Rhythm. 2020;**17**(2):184-189

[23] Wielandts JY, Kyriakopoulou M, Almorad A, Hilfiker G, Strisciuglio T, Phlips T, et al. Prospective randomized evaluation of high power during CLOSE-guided pulmonary vein isolation: The POWER-AF study. Circulation. Arrhythmia and Electrophysiology. 2021;**14**(1):e009112

[24] Ravi V, Poudyal A, Abid QU, Larsen T, Krishnan K, Sharma PS, et al. High-power short duration vs. conventional radiofrequency ablation of atrial fibrillation: A systematic review and meta-analysis. Europace. 2021;**23**(5):710-721

[25] Blockhaus C, Muller P, Vom Dahl S, Leonhardt S, Haussinger D, Gerguri S, et al. Low incidence of esophageal lesions after pulmonary vein isolation using contact-force sensing catheter without esophageal temperature probe. International Heart Journal. 2017;**58**(6):880-884

[26] Yarlagadda B, Deneke T, Turagam M, Dar T, Paleti S, Parikh V, et al. Temporal relationships between

esophageal injury type and progression in patients undergoing atrial fibrillation catheter ablation. Heart Rhythm. 2019;**16**(2):204-212

[27] Wolf M, El Haddad M, De Wilde V, Phlips T, De Pooter J, Almorad A, et al. Endoscopic evaluation of the esophagus after catheter ablation of atrial fibrillation using contiguous and optimized radiofrequency applications. Heart Rhythm. 2019;**16**(7):1013-1020

[28] Kaneshiro T, Kamioka M, Hijioka N, Yamada S, Yokokawa T, Misaka T, et al. Characteristics of esophageal injury in ablation of atrial fibrillation using a high-power short-duration setting. Circulation. Arrhythmia and Electrophysiology. 2020;**13**(10):e008602

[29] Vassallo F, Meigre LL, Serpa E, Cunha CL, Carloni H, Simoes A Jr, et al. Reduced esophageal heating in high-power short-duration atrial fibrillation ablation in the contact force catheter era. Pacing and Clinical Electrophysiology. 2021;**44**(7):1185-1192

[30] Kottmaier M, Popa M, Bourier F, Reents T, Cifuentes J, Semmler V, et al. Safety and outcome of very high-power short-duration ablation using 70 W for pulmonary vein isolation in patients with paroxysmal atrial fibrillation. Europace. 2020;**22**(3):388-393

[31] Reddy VY, Grimaldi M, De Potter T, Vijgen JM, Bulava A, Duytschaever MF, et al. Pulmonary vein isolation with very high power, short duration, temperature-controlled lesions: The QDOT-FAST trial. JACC: Clinical Electrophysiology. 2019;**5**(7):778-786

Chapter 7

Epicardial Radiofrequency Ablation: Who, When, and How?

Chin-Yu Lin

Abstract

In the past decades, it has been known that reentry circuits for ventricular tachycardia or focal triggers of premature ventricular complexes are not limited to the subendocardial myocardium. Rather, intramural or subepicardial substrates may also give rise to ventricular tachycardia, particularly in those with non-ischemic cardiomyopathy. Besides, some of the idiopathic ventricular tachycardia might be originated from epicardial foci. Percutaneous epicardial mapping and ablation have been successfully introduced to treat this sub-epicardiac ventricular tachycardia. Herein, this chapter reviews the indications for epicardial ablation and the identification of epicardial ventricular tachycardia by disease entity, electrocardiography and imaging modalities. This chapter also described the optimal technique for epicardial access and the potential complication.

Keywords: epicardial, ventricular tachycardia, ablation, non-ischemic cardiomyopathy, idiopathic

1. Introduction

The pericardium is a two-layer membrane surrounding the heart and vital vessels. The two-layer structure included a serous visceral membrane inside and a fibrous membrane (parietal pericardium) outside. The fibrous membrane is adhered to the diaphragm, posterior part of sternum by the tissue and ligament to fix the heart. The pericardium encloses the heart and pericardial fluid, which provides lubrication for the myocardium [1]. Pericardial puncture is a standard and useful therapeutic procedure for the treatment of diagnosis of tamponade or symptomatic pericardial effusion [1]. In 1996, Sosa et al. first described the use of pericardial puncture in an electrophysiological laboratory for epicardial ablation in ventricular arrhythmia, [2] the use of pericardial puncture to map and ablate ventricular arrhythmia started to expand in other diseases [3].

Before to the era of catheter ablation with epicardial approach, patients with ventricular tachycardia (VT) refractory to catheter ablation from the endocardium often required surgical approach. The technique became well-developed and skilled in high-volume center recently. Many centers reported the successful application of the epicedial ablation in a diverse range of cardiac arrhythmia. Therefore, the indication for the epicardial approach has extended. The potential indication included substrate/ idiopathic VTs, accessory pathways, and miscellaneous supraventricular tachycardias [4]. Since Sosa et al. first introduced the application of epicardial ablation for the ventricular arrhythmias (VAs) in Chagas disease, [2] the use of this technique through a percutaneous method has been applied to other diseases [3].

In the patients with ischemic cardiomyopathy due to prior myocardial infarction (MI) and VT, the involved circuit mostly involved the inner part of the heart [5]. In the previous report, part of the ischemic VT circuit may involve areas within the subepicardial area [6]. The advantage of the epicardial approach was demonstrated by clinical study. An approach with combined endo-epicardial mapping/ablation has been reported to show a better outcome selected patients with non-ischemic cardiomyopathy (NICM) VT ischemic VT [7–10]. Furthermore, the percutaneous technique for epicardial access have been proven to improve outcomes with an acceptable risk of peri-operative adverse event in experienced operator or high-volume centers [11]. However, there were many surrounding epicardial vascular structures or nerves in the tract of epicardial puncture. The unskilled operators may encounter serious and detrimental complications. Prior studies have reported the incidence rate of major complications around 4.1-8.8%, including adverse event of a hemopericardium, intra-abdominal bleeding, and arterial/venous/nerve injuries [11–14]. This chapter was aimed to discuss the clinical implication, patient selection, and detailed procedure for the epicardial ablation in the patients with VA.

2. Who should be considered to perform the epicardial approach?

2.1 Contraindication for endocardial approach

Generally, the endocardial approach was contraindicated in the following condition

1. Endocardial mural thrombus was presented.

2. Coexisted mechanical valves were presented in the mitral and aortic valve

In the patient with the presence of newly-identified mural thrombus, the strategy of endocardial ablation should be postponed. Previous report described the results of endocardial VT ablation in 8 patients with identified old thrombus [15]. Intracardiac echocardiography (ICE) seems to be more sensitive for the detection of LV thrombi compared to transthoracic echocardiography (TTE) and is helpful in real-time navigation of the mapping / ablation catheter. No procedural or periprocedural complications were observed in this retrospective study [15].

Mechanical prosthetic aortic and mitral valves preclude either a retrograde aortic or transseptal approach to the left ventricle (LV) endocardium. Several operators have reported previously on the use of unconventional techniques during VT ablation such as transventricular septal puncture, [16, 17] epicardial approach, [18] transmechanical valve approach, [19] transcoronary venous approach, [20] or transapical approach [21].

2.2 Contraindication for percutaneous epicardial approach

Intrapericardial access is usually obtained through a subxiphoidal pericardial puncture. This approach might not be possible in patients with pericardial adhesions caused by prior cardiac surgery, pericarditis, or prior epicardial ablation. (**Figures 1** and **2**) In such cases, a hybrid procedure involving surgical access to

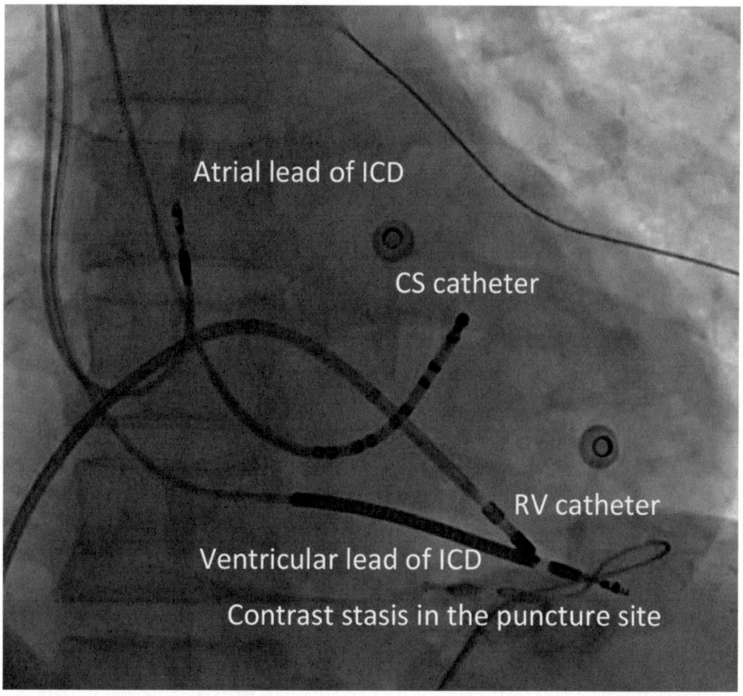

Figure 1.
Epicardial puncture in a patient with prior epicardial ablation. The figure showed the anterior–posterior view during epicardial puncture. The fluoroscopic view demonstrated the contrast stasis in the bottom of the epicardium due to prior ablation and severe adhesion. The wire could not advance further in the localized epicardial space.

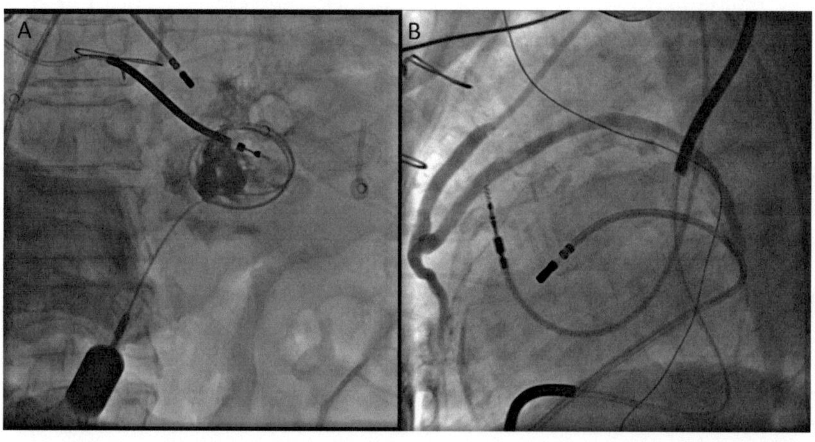

Figure 2.
Epicardial puncture in a patient with prior coronary artery bypass grafting. The figure showed the anterior–posterior view during after an initial puncture. The fluoroscopic view demonstrated the contrast stasis in the bottom of the epicardium due to prior cardiac surgery severe adhesion. The wire could not advance further in the localized epicardial space (panel A). After several attempts, the ablation catheter was advanced to the limited epicardial space. Coronary angiography was done before the ablation to avoid coronary injury through the graft (panel B).

a subxiphoid pericardial window or lateral thoracotomy might be a feasible and safe method of performing epicardial catheter ablation in the electrophysiology laboratory [4].

2.3 Endocardial approaches were more favorable than epicardial approach

2.3.1 Myocardial infarction related VT

The previous study showed a good response with subendocardial resection to treat the subendocardial location of the VT substrate from surgical experience, which indicated the endocardial VT circuits [22]. Furthermore, the endocardial catheter ablation with mappable VT demonstrated good acute procedural success rate. However, the long-term outcome was unsatisfied [23]. A prior study examined all ischemic cardiomyopathy (ICM) VT cases with endocardial and/or epicardial mapping/ablation. Epicardial approach was applied in 14% of patients, and application of ablation in the epicardium was done in 8.5% patients. Part of the patient (0.5%) did not undergo epicardial ablation because of proximity to an epicardial coronary artery to the of identifying epicardial substrate [24]. In an Asian study from Taiwan, the epicardial approach for the ICM-related VT was rarely reported [14]. This may be related to the highest quality and convenience of Taiwan's public health system. A recent non-randomized study provided evidence of epicardial-endocardial approach in these patients [25]. Generally, the region of myocardial infarction does not appear to be predictive of epicardial involvement. On the other hand, imaging, such as cardiac magnetic resonance imaging (MRI), cardiac computed tomography, or nuclear scintigraphy suggesting transmural infarction may identify patients more likely to have epicardial substrate [26].

2.3.2 Idiopathic ventricular arrhythmia

The recent review article summarized most common idiopathic VT arising from the right and left ventricle: (1) outflow tract VT, (2) fascicular VT, (3) intracavitary VT, (4) perivalvular VT, and (5) epicardial VT [27]. Around 1. 8–9. 2% of idiopathic VT were raised from the epicardium. In the prior study, the electrocardiography is a useful parameter for predicting the successful ablation sites of VT originating from the continuum between the aortic sinus of Valsalva (ASV) and the left ventricle (LV) summit [28]. In the results, aVL/aVR Q-wave ratio is useful in the prediction of successful ablation sites. A coronary venous approach / pericardial access might be required with a cutoff value of 1.536-1.740 and > 1.740 respectively.

2.4 Epicardial approaches were more favorable than endocardial approach

2.4.1 Brugada syndrome catheter ablation

Brugada syndrome (BrS) is one of the main causes of sudden cardiac arrest in young population [29]. The efficacy and adverse effects of anti-arrhythmic drugs on BrS was disappointing. Catheter ablation emerged and offers an alternative therapeutic strategy for these patients with repeat recurrent implantable cardioverter defibrillator (ICD) shock after the ICD implantation. Nademanee et al. first demonstrated the effectiveness and safety of ablating the arrhythmogenic electrogram at the epicardium of right ventricular outflow tract (RVOT) to decrease the VT/VF burden [30]. Further study on the post-mortem heart demonstrated interstitial fibrosis and reduced gap junction expression in the epicardium of RVOT in BrS patients. The abnormal fibrosis resulted in arrhythmogenic potentials. Eliminating the arrhythmogenic potentials by using ablation could abolish the BrS ECG pattern and reduce VT/VF burden. In the clinical practice, the operator may perform

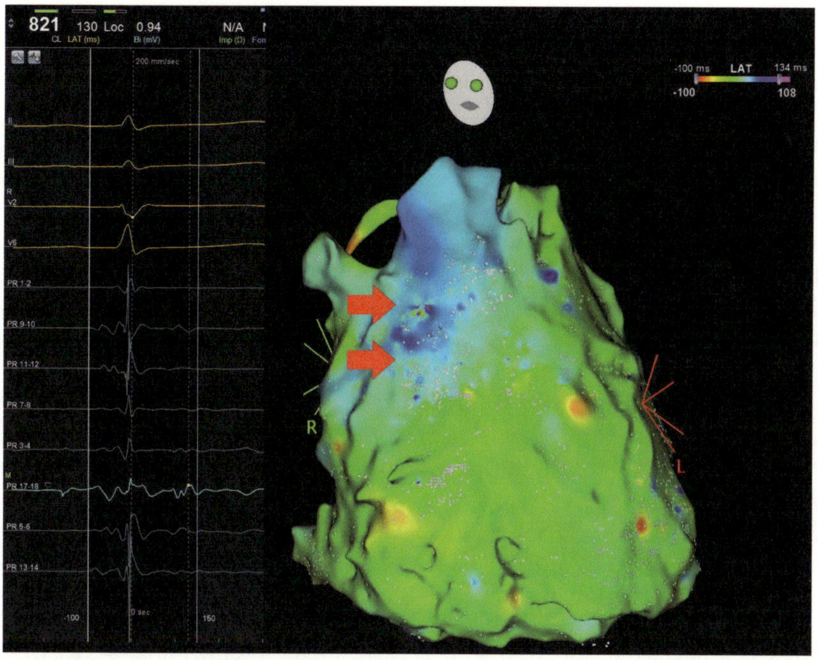

Figure 3.
Local fractioned potential in the epicardial right ventricular outflow tract of a patient with Brugada syndrome. The left panel demonstrated local abnormal signal and delayed electrogram, which was localized in the epicardial right ventricular outflow tract. (red arrow, right panel) this patient was diagnosed as Brugada syndrome and survived from an episode of sudden cardiac death due to ventricular fibrillation.

epicardial mapping and identified the slow conduction zone and abnormal electrogram in the RV epicardially. (**Figure 3**) The electrophysiological group in Taipei Veterans General Hospital first introduced the warm water instillation, which would enhance the phenotype and functional substrate in the patient with BrS. Ablation by targeting the triggers and abnormal epicardial substrates provided an effective strategy for preventing ventricular tachyarrhythmia recurrences in BrS [31].

2.4.2 Arrhythmogenic right ventricular cardiomyopathy

Arrhythmogenic right ventricular cardiomyopathy (ARVC) is a heritable desmosome disorder. The clinical manifestations vary from asymptomatic concealed stage, electrical abnormality with ventricular arrhythmias (VAs), to progressive heart failure [32, 33]. Catheter ablation is emerging as an alternative therapy for drug-refractory VAs in patients with ARVC. Although the catheter ablation could result in acute procedural success with VT termination, the high incidence of recurrence limited the role of ablation in ARVC initially [34, 35]. The application of epicardial and endocardial ablation of VT in the patients with ARVC had been proposed with good effects acute and long-term outcome and VAs-freedom [36, 37]. Recent studies also demonstrated that 45 ~ 84. 6% patients were free from VA recurrences or ICD therapy through the combination of endocardial and epicardial ablation [38, 39]. Epicardial approach is required in more than one third ARVC patients for achieving non-inducibility in the prior reports [40]. The number of fulfilled SAECG criteria was correlated to the extent of diseased epicardial substrate and could be a potential surrogate marker to predict the requirement of epicardial ablation in ARVC with drug-refractory VA [40].

2.4.3 Non-ischemic cardiomyopathy

In contrast to ischemic cardiomyopathy, non-ischemic cardiomyopathy (NICM) consists of a heterogeneous group of diseases [41] affecting the myocardium. Despite the progress and improvement in the pharmacological medication of heart failure in recent decades have significantly decreased the disease progression and mortality in NICM patients, anti-arrhythmic medications and ICD implantations remain the most important treatment for patients carrying a high risk of VT/VF or who have experienced aborted SCD due to fatal VT/VF [42]. Owing to the improvement in electro-anatomic mapping and ablation catheter, catheter ablation of VT in NICM patients has been recognized as an upcoming issue [43]. A prior study proven the promising results that a successful catheter ablation could reduce VT recurrences and improve the survival in NICM patients regardless of the functional class status or left ventricular function [44]. NICM VTs in different disease entities could result from non-uniform arrhythmogenic substrates, which can lead to different ablation outcomes.

With the exception of ARVC and BrS, the arrhythmogenic substrates in NICM that could be identified by electroanatomic mapping, are mostly located in the base or perivalvular region of the LV, which is distinct from the substrate ICM [45]. The arrhythmogenic potentials could be identified from the endocardial/epicardial aspect in the patients with NICM [46]. These arrhythmogenic substrates frequently associate fibrosis tissue that leads to conduction disturbance and fractionated electrograms [47]. Aside from the electroanatomic substrate mapping with bipolar/unipolar voltage, cardiac MR can provide additional information to unmask the scar distribution as a non-invasive manner [48–50]. Additionally, patients with scar involving the inferolateral aspect of the LV, which frequently requires an epicardial approach, usually have a better prognosis than those with anteroseptal scar [51].

A comprehensive investigation of patients with NICM and VT includes cardiac imaging and genetic testing. These information might enable recognition of undiagnosed diseases, such as isolated and active cardiac sarcoidosis or inherited cardiomyopathies. An accurate diagnosis could improve patient selection for ablation and early consideration of individualized treatments [52].

3. When should be considered to perform the epicardial approach?

An epicardial approach could performed for patients with refractory ablation from an endocardial approach. The clinical documentation of surface ECG could provide specific electrocardiographies evidence supporting an epicardial origin [28, 53, 54]. In cases with a disease entity favoring an epicardial substrate, or those with electroanatomic mapping supporting the existence of a diseased epicardial substrate, an epicardial approach could be considered [30, 55, 56].

Before preparing for epicardial approach, the first step is to localize the VT origin and identify the potential regions of arrhythmogenic substrates. The surface ECG morphologies provide the information about the origin and the potential need for an epicardial approach [53]. Standardized echocardiography or intracardiac could delineate the valvular structure, area of hypokinesia or akinesia, and excluding any intracardiac thrombus [57]. Computed tomography (CT) and cardiac MRI with a late gadolinium enhancement, could localize the regions of abnormal tissue in specific protocol [48–50]. The distribution and extent of the scar is useful for deciding the ablation strategy, such as an epicardial approach, transcoronary venous ablation,

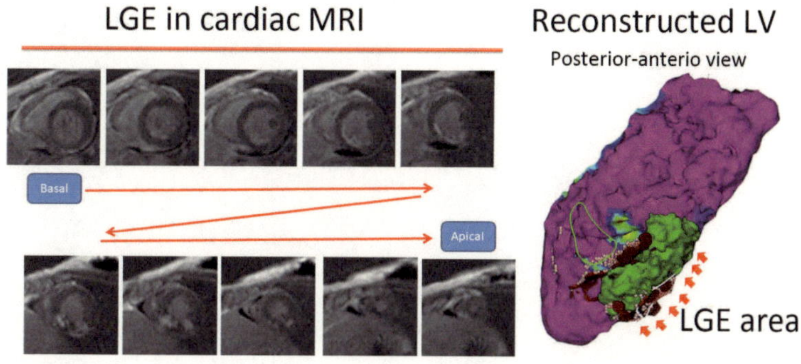

Figure 4.
Cardiac magnetic resonance imaging (CMRI) and three-dimensional reconstruction in a patient with non-ischemic myocardial infarction. The CMRI demonstrated a late gadolinium enhancement (LGE) in the mid posterior wall. The three-dimensional reconstruction was performed to guide the catheter ablation.

alcohol ablation, or simultaneous bipolar ablation. The integration of the reconstructed images obtained from CT and MRI and 3-D navigation, mapping systems (**Figure 4**) can aid in the illustration of the structural complexity and avoidance of damage to the critical regions, in terms of vascular or nervous structures.

4. How to perform the epicardial approach?

4.1 Traditional method (posterior approach)

After obtaining informed consent, the procedure would be performed with the patients in a fasting state under general anesthesia. Pre-procedure subxiphoid echocardiography was recommended to perform routinely. In some cases, the echocardiography could help the operator avoid liver or gastric injuries. A subxiphoid puncture was performed to penetrate the pericardium in the inferior aspect of the hear according to the technique described by Sosa et al [2]. Access to the pericardium was achieved by using an 18 G Tuohy Needle (Arrow International, Inc., Reading, PA, USA) in the laboratory of Taipei Veterans General Hospital through the subxiphoid process. The anteroposterior projection was usually used to direct the access in the anterior/posterior plane, while the left anterior oblique (LAO) 60° projection was used to guide the needle leftward tangentially to the cardiac border. **Figure 5** demonstrated the adjacent structure with these two views by reconstruction of the CT. After passing through the diaphragm, 1-2 cm^3 of contrast could be injected between the diaphragm and pericardium to observe tenting of the pericardium. After entering the posterior side of pericardium, a 0.032 guidewire would be advanced to the left heart border in the LAO projection, and 10 cm^3 of contrast could be injected into the pericardial space through a 5F dilator or the side hole of a 5Fr sheath to allow for visualization of any adhesions. (**Figure 6**) An 8-Fr Sheath or flexible long Sheath would be exchanged by using the guide wire. The ablation/mapping catheter would be inserted through the sheath after obtain the access to avoid injury by the edge of the sheath. Angiography would be performed while locating the catheter in the interested area to avoid coronary injury. (**Figure 7**) After the procedure, the epicardial sheath was exchanged for a pigtail. Pericardial injections of hydrocortisone 100 mg and ketorolac tromethamine 30 mg were routinely given immediately and 24 hours after the epicardial procedure to prevent any future epicardial adhesions or pericarditis.

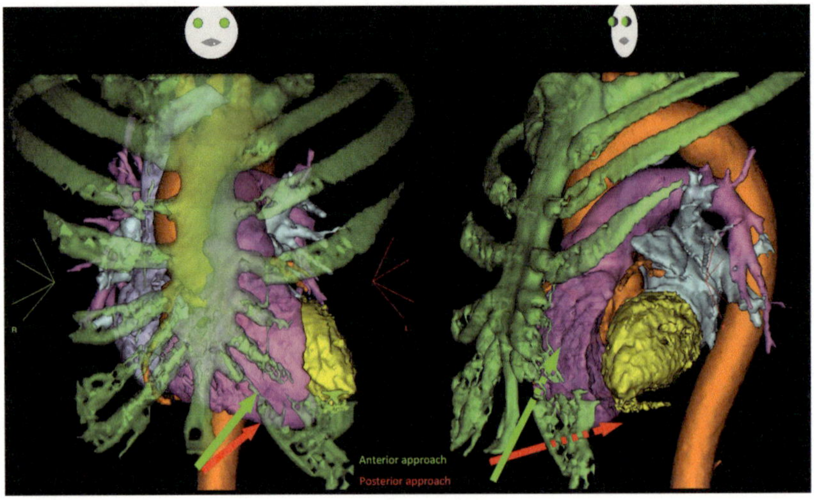

Figure 5.
The anatomy with anterior–posterior view (left panel) and LAO view (right panel). The green arrow indicated the anterior approach and the red arrow indicated the posterior approach.

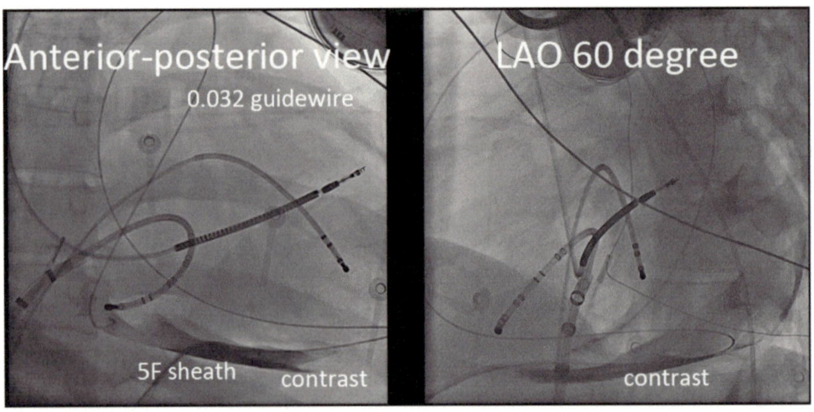

Figure 6.
Epicardial puncture in a patient with arrhythmogenic right ventricular cardiomyopathy. The anterior–posterior view (left panel) and LAO view (right panel) showed the wire in the epicardial space surrounding the whole heart and the contrast in the epicardial space without adhesion.

4.2 Needle-in-needle method

A 'needle-in-needle' technique for epicardial access has been described by Kumar et al [58]. In this approach, a 7-cm 18-gauge needle is inserted beneath the sternum. The purpose of this short needle is to provide stability and tactile feedback for a long (15- or 20-cm) micropuncture 21-gauge needle, which is inserted through the 18-gauge needle. Once the 21-gauge needle is inserted into the pericardial space, along 0.018-inch guidewire with a floppy tip is advanced into the pericardial space. Upon fluoroscopic confirmation that the guide wire has been inserted into the pericardium both needles are then removed. Micropuncture dilators are then used to upsize the guide wire to a 0.35-inch wire and ultimately, an 8-Fr sheath is introduced into the pericardial space. The 'needle-in-needle' approach was compared to the traditional methods. Successful epicardial access was achieved in 100% of the 'needle-in-needle' cases, as compared to 94% with the Sosa technique. Failure of epicardial access in the traditional method were due to prior cardiac surgery [13] or

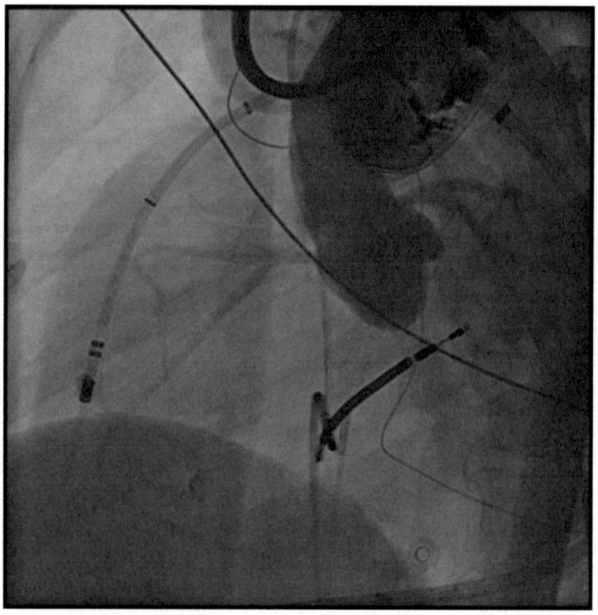

Figure 7.
Angiography before epicardial ablation. After a successful epicardial puncture through posterior approach, the angiography was performed before the ablation to avoid coronary injury.

adhesions from prior epicardial mapping/ablation or episodes of pericarditis [7]. Major pericardial bleeding was similar between both techniques [58].

4.3 Anterior approach vs. posterior approach

In anatomic, there is a potential space below the sternum and xyphoid process. While puncturing below the xyphoid process, the needle might directly pass through the fibrous pericardium avoiding the puncture through the diaphragm [59]. The term of "anterior approach" was used for the epicardial approach via this potential space (**Figure 8**). This approach was based on the previous finding that an increased fluid in the anterior part of the heart during supine position [60, 61]. Theoretically, the density of myocardium is heavier than and pericardial fluid. During supine position, the heart might force the pericardial fluid to the anterior part within the pericardium. Keramati et al. reported the anterior approach was successfully performed in 100% of patients in their study cohort [62]. The success rate was similar between the anterior approach and the needle in needle approach. On the other hand, the success rate of the anterior approach was higher than the traditional approach. In the report, there were no major pericardial hemorrhage and even the PV puncture. **Figure 9** demonstrated the illustration of the anterior approach and posterior approach.

4.4 Fluoroscopic approach with carbon dioxide insufflation

The technique of carbon dioxide insufflation was first reported with right atrial exit in human study by Greenbaum et al [63]. A modified approach with exit from the coronary sinus was reported by Silberbauer et al [64]. The pericardial space was insufflated with carbon dioxide after creating the exit, which allowing visualization of the pericardial membrane and separated membrane to the myocardium. The epicardial space with carbon dioxide allowed safe epicardial puncture and minimized the risk of RV perforation. A multi-center registry was conducted with

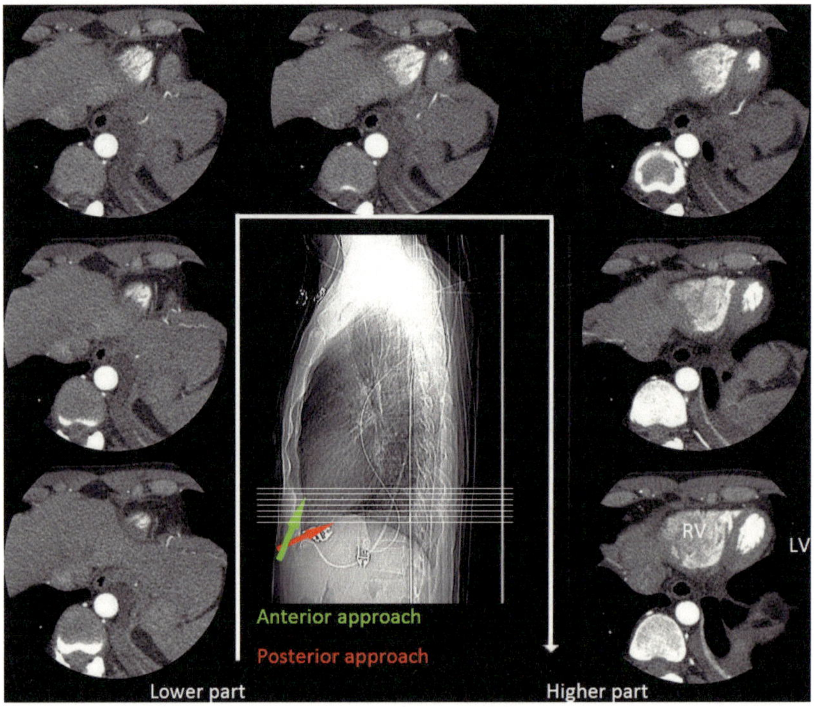

Figure 8.
An illustration of anterior and posterior approach. The figure showed the X-ray from the lateral view. The green arrow indicated the anterior approach and the red arrow indicated the posterior approach. The horizontal cut of the hears from lower caudal part of the cranial part. The white arrow indicates the sequence from the lower part of the higher part. Each cut was corresponding to the horizontal while line in the X-ray.

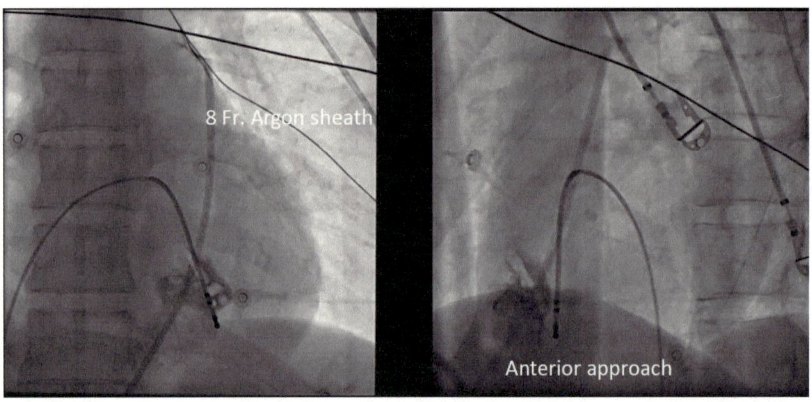

Figure 9.
Example of anterior approach. Anterior approach was performed successfully. The guide wire was exchanged with an 8 Fr sheath after confirming the location.

this modified approach. There was no patient complicated with the RV puncture of coronary artery injury [65]. However, the operator needs to take care of the potential risk of bleeding from the exit site.

4.5 Wire-guided puncture

This approach was first described by Long et al [64] in 2019. This approach was different from traditional approach using the contrast-filled syringe to the needle.

In the wire-guided approach, a J-tipped guide wire is within the needle during puncture. After advancing the needle the adjacent area of the pericardium, the wire was advanced. The wire would curve back if it reached the parietal pericardium, and the operator could feel the heart pulsations. The wire was dragged back to the needle's tip at this point. The wire and needle were both pressed again at the same time. While the needle was traveling through the epicardium, the wire would fall into the pericardial region. The study found that this method was safe and that the success rate was comparable to that of the traditional method.

4.6 Surgical access

Pericardial window provides clear visualization of the epicardial myocardium and manipulation of the mapping catheter and Realtime feedback for the location of the mapping catheter cooperating with the 3-D anatomic mapping system. The operator might not able to perform percutaneous subxiphoid access in patients with pericardial adhesions. In these patients, a surgical window may be required to gain access to the pericardium. This technique involves a subxiphoid incision, followed by manual lysis of adhesions to visualize the epicardial surface. A sheath was then placed into the pericardial space after opening a small window in the pericardium [66]. This technique should be considered in patients with a prior history of cardiac surgery with dense pericardial adhesions [67].

5. Periprocedural complications of an epicardial approach

In the prior report, the incidence of major complications was 10.0%, and that for minor complications was 17.5% [14]. Prior single and multicenter studies also reported similar findings [11, 12]. However, it is important to keep in mind that these complication rates were obtained from arrhythmia centers with an experience of epicardial approach. The surgical backup was required for potential major complications. Major complications of intra-abdominal bleeding due to vessel damage and MI owing to ablation in the adjacent area were reported [68]. Another possible cause of intra-abdominal bleeding is the liver puncture or perforation. The operator should also take care for the location of the coronary sinus. Coronary sinus puncture might occur if the puncture site is close to the base of the heart. Thus, detailed preoperative evaluations by ECG, echocardiography, and peri-operative image, especially for patients with hepatomegaly or a congested liver, may prevent the occurrence of any life-threatening complications.

RV puncture was not uncommon and it has been reported to be a minor complication with an incidence of 4. 5 ~ 7. 5% [13, 14, 68]. The RV puncture could be reduced after a learning curve. Post-procedural pericarditis was common. Prolonged and intolerable chest pain due to pericarditis might be improved by the administration of intrapericardial steroids and non-steroidal anti-inflammatory drugs. Phrenic nerve injuries and coronary artery damage could be avoided by phrenic nerve pacing and pre-ablation angiography [69, 70].

5.1 Patients with anticoagulant

In the patient with anticoagulant, the epicardial access could be performed according to the guideline. After excluding the potential risk of adhesion, history of epicardial surgery, and complex anatomy, the procedure might be classified as a minor risk procedure in an experienced operator [71]. Therefore, the procedure could be performed at NOAC through level (12 or 24 hours after the first intake) and resume after the procedure or latest next day without active bleeding. Beside, the procedure should be better performed by experienced operator and avoid repeated RV puncture. Antidote or blood transfusion should be available in the hospital.

6. Conclusion

The need for an epicardial approach for VA ablation displayed a gradually increasing trend. The disease entity, prior surgery or ablation, electrocardiography, image study, and other diagnostic test should be carefully reviewed before the decision making. The prior studies demonstrate the effectiveness of epicardial catheter ablation with acceptable safety in experienced referral center.

Acknowledgements

This work was supported by Ministry of Science and Technology of Taiwan (109-2314-B-075 -076 -MY3), Grant of TVGH (V109B-013).

This work was contributed to the electrophysiological team in Taipei Veterans General Hospital.

The **Figure 5** was contributed to the Mr. Liu, Kuan-Hong from Johnson & Johnson.

Conflict of interest

The author declares no conflict of interest.

Author details

Chin-Yu Lin[1,2]

1 Institute of Clinical Medicine, and Cardiovascular Research Center, National Yang Ming Chiao Tung University, Taiwan

2 Division of Cardiology, Department of Medicine, Taipei Veterans General Hospital, Taipei, Taiwan

*Address all correspondence to: clouaa@gmail.com

References

[1] Adler, Y., et al., *2015 ESC Guidelines for the diagnosis and management of pericardial diseases: The Task Force for the Diagnosis and Management of Pericardial Diseases of the European Society of Cardiology (ESC)Endorsed by: The European Association for Cardio-Thoracic Surgery (EACTS).* Eur Heart J, 2015. **36**(42): p. 2921-2964.

[2] Sosa, E., et al., *A new technique to perform epicardial mapping in the electrophysiology laboratory.* J Cardiovasc Electrophysiol, 1996. **7**(6): p. 531-6.

[3] Boyle, N.G. and K. Shivkumar, *Epicardial interventions in electrophysiology.* Circulation, 2012. **126**(14): p. 1752-69.

[4] Yamada, T., *Transthoracic epicardial catheter ablation: indications, techniques, and complications.* Circ J, 2013. **77**(7): p. 1672-80.

[5] Aliot, E.M., et al., *EHRA/HRS Expert Consensus on Catheter Ablation of Ventricular Arrhythmias: developed in a partnership with the European Heart Rhythm Association (EHRA), a Registered Branch of the European Society of Cardiology (ESC), and the Heart Rhythm Society (HRS); in collaboration with the American College of Cardiology (ACC) and the American Heart Association (AHA).* Europace, 2009. **11**(6): p. 771-817.

[6] Svenson, R.H., et al., *Termination of ventricular tachycardia with epicardial laser photocoagulation: a clinical comparison with patients undergoing successful endocardial photocoagulation alone.* J Am Coll Cardiol, 1990. **15**(1): p. 163-70.

[7] Sosa, E., et al., *Nonsurgical transthoracic epicardial catheter ablation to treat recurrent ventricular tachycardia occurring late after myocardial infarction.* J Am Coll Cardiol, 2000. **35**(6): p. 1442-9.

[8] Maury, P., et al., *Histopathologic effects of endocardial and epicardial percutaneous radiofrequency catheter ablation in dilated nonischemic cardiomyopathy.* Pacing Clin Electrophysiol, 2008. **31**(9): p. 1218-22.

[9] Cano, O., et al., *Electroanatomic substrate and ablation outcome for suspected epicardial ventricular tachycardia in left ventricular nonischemic cardiomyopathy.* J Am Coll Cardiol, 2009. **54**(9): p. 799-808.

[10] Santangeli, P., et al., *Long-Term Outcome With Catheter Ablation of Ventricular Tachycardia in Patients With Arrhythmogenic Right Ventricular Cardiomyopathy.* Circ Arrhythm Electrophysiol, 2015. **8**(6): p. 1413-21.

[11] Della Bella, P., et al., *Epicardial ablation for ventricular tachycardia: a European multicenter study.* Circ Arrhythm Electrophysiol, 2011. **4**(5): p. 653-9.

[12] Tung, R., et al., *Epicardial ablation of ventricular tachycardia: an institutional experience of safety and efficacy.* Heart Rhythm, 2013. **10**(4): p. 490-8.

[13] Sacher, F., et al., *Epicardial ventricular tachycardia ablation a multicenter safety study.* J Am Coll Cardiol, 2010. **55**(21): p. 2366-72.

[14] Lin, C.Y., et al., *Safety and Efficacy of Epicardial Ablation of Ventricular Tachyarrhythmias: Experience from a Tertiary Referral Center in Taiwan.* Acta Cardiol Sin, 2018. **34**(1): p. 49-58.

[15] Peichl, P., et al., *Catheter Ablation of Ventricular Tachycardia in the Presence of an Old Endocavitary Thrombus Guided by Intracardiac Echocardiography.* Pacing Clin Electrophysiol, 2016. **39**(6): p. 581-7.

[16] Vaseghi, M., et al., *Percutaneous interventricular septal access in a patient*

with aortic and mitral mechanical valves: a novel technique for catheter ablation of ventricular tachycardia. Heart Rhythm, 2013. **10**(7): p. 1069-73.

[17] Santangeli, P., G.C. Shaw, and F.E. Marchlinski, *Radiofrequency Wire Facilitated Interventricular Septal Access for Catheter Ablation of Ventricular Tachycardia in a Patient With Aortic and Mitral Mechanical Valves.* Circ Arrhythm Electrophysiol, 2017. **10**(1).

[18] Soejima, K., et al., *Epicardial catheter ablation of ventricular tachycardia in no entry left ventricle: mechanical aortic and mitral valves.* Circ Arrhythm Electrophysiol, 2015. **8**(2): p. 381-9.

[19] Herweg, B., et al., *Ablation of left ventricular tachycardia via transeptal approach and crossing of a mechanical mitral valve prosthesis.* Pacing Clin Electrophysiol, 2010. **33**(7): p. 900-3.

[20] Najjar, J., et al., *Radiofrequency ablation of an epicardial ventricular tachycardia through the great cardiac vein in a patient with mitro-aortic mechanical prostheses.* Europace, 2007. **9**(11): p. 1069-72.

[21] Vurgun, V.K., et al., *Percutaneous transapical approach and transcatheter closure for ventricular tachycardia ablation.* Pacing Clin Electrophysiol, 2018. **41**(3): p. 334-337.

[22] Miller, J.M., et al., *Subendocardial resection for ventricular tachycardia: predictors of surgical success.* Circulation, 1984. **70**(4): p. 624-31.

[23] Almendral, J. and M.E. Josephson, *All patients with hemodynamically tolerated postinfarction ventricular tachycardia do not require an implantable cardioverter-defibrillator.* Circulation, 2007. **116**(10): p. 1204-12.

[24] Sarkozy, A., et al., *Epicardial ablation of ventricular tachycardia in ischemic heart disease.* Circ Arrhythm Electrophysiol, 2013. **6**(6): p. 1115-22.

[25] Izquierdo, M., et al., *Endo-epicardial versus only-endocardial ablation as a first line strategy for the treatment of ventricular tachycardia in patients with ischemic heart disease.* Circ Arrhythm Electrophysiol, 2015. **8**(4): p. 882-9.

[26] Acosta, J., et al., *Infarct transmurality as a criterion for first-line endo-epicardial substrate-guided ventricular tachycardia ablation in ischemic cardiomyopathy.* Heart Rhythm, 2016. **13**(1): p. 85-95.

[27] Tanawuttiwat, T., S. Nazarian, and H. Calkins, *The role of catheter ablation in the management of ventricular tachycardia.* Eur Heart J, 2016. **37**(7): p. 594-609.

[28] Lin, C.Y., et al., *Radiofrequency catheter ablation of ventricular arrhythmias originating from the continuum between the aortic sinus of Valsalva and the left ventricular summit: Electrocardiographic characteristics and correlative anatomy.* Heart Rhythm, 2016. **13**(1): p. 111-21.

[29] Vohra, J., S. Rajagopalan, and C.G.C.W. Group, *Update on the Diagnosis and Management of Brugada Syndrome.* Heart Lung Circ, 2015. **24**(12): p. 1141-8.

[30] Nademanee, K., et al., *Prevention of ventricular fibrillation episodes in Brugada syndrome by catheter ablation over the anterior right ventricular outflow tract epicardium.* Circulation, 2011. **123**(12): p. 1270-9.

[31] Chung, F.P., et al., *A novel method to enhance phenotype, epicardial functional substrates, and ventricular tachyarrhythmias in Brugada syndrome.* Heart Rhythm, 2017. **14**(4): p. 508-517.

[32] te Riele, A.S., et al., *Yield of serial evaluation in at-risk family members of patients with ARVD/C.* J Am Coll Cardiol, 2014. **64**(3): p. 293-301.

[33] Mast, T.P., et al., *Right Ventricular Imaging and Computer Simulation for Electromechanical Substrate Characterization in Arrhythmogenic Right Ventricular Cardiomyopathy.* J Am Coll Cardiol, 2016. **68**(20): p. 2185-2197.

[34] Verma, A., et al., *Short- and long-term success of substrate-based mapping and ablation of ventricular tachycardia in arrhythmogenic right ventricular dysplasia.* Circulation, 2005. **111**(24): p. 3209-16.

[35] Dalal, D., et al., *Long-term efficacy of catheter ablation of ventricular tachycardia in patients with arrhythmogenic right ventricular dysplasia/cardiomyopathy.* J Am Coll Cardiol, 2007. **50**(5): p. 432-40.

[36] Garcia, F.C., et al., *Epicardial substrate and outcome with epicardial ablation of ventricular tachycardia in arrhythmogenic right ventricular cardiomyopathy/dysplasia.* Circulation, 2009. **120**(5): p. 366-75.

[37] Lin, C.Y., et al., *Characteristics of recurrent ventricular tachyarrhythmia after catheter ablation in patients with arrhythmogenic right ventricular cardiomyopathy.* J Cardiovasc Electrophysiol, 2019. **30**(4): p. 582-592.

[38] Bai, R., et al., *Ablation of ventricular arrhythmias in arrhythmogenic right ventricular dysplasia/cardiomyopathy: arrhythmia-free survival after endo-epicardial substrate based mapping and ablation.* Circ Arrhythm Electrophysiol, 2011. **4**(4): p. 478-85.

[39] Philips, B., et al., *Outcomes of catheter ablation of ventricular tachycardia in arrhythmogenic right ventricular dysplasia/cardiomyopathy.* Circ Arrhythm Electrophysiol, 2012. **5**(3): p. 499-505.

[40] Chung, F.P., et al., *Application of noninvasive signal-averaged electrocardiogram analysis in predicting the requirement of epicardial ablation in patients with arrhythmogenic right ventricular cardiomyopathy.* Heart Rhythm, 2020. **17**(4): p. 584-591.

[41] Wu, A.H., *Management of patients with non-ischaemic cardiomyopathy.* Heart, 2007. **93**(3): p. 403-8.

[42] Pedersen, C.T., et al., *EHRA/HRS/APHRS expert consensus on ventricular arrhythmias.* Heart Rhythm, 2014. **11**(10): p. e166-96.

[43] Sacher, F., et al., *Ventricular tachycardia ablation: evolution of patients and procedures over 8 years.* Circ Arrhythm Electrophysiol, 2008. **1**(3): p. 153-61.

[44] Tung, R., et al., *Freedom from recurrent ventricular tachycardia after catheter ablation is associated with improved survival in patients with structural heart disease: An International VT Ablation Center Collaborative Group study.* Heart Rhythm, 2015. **12**(9): p. 1997-2007.

[45] Hsia, H.H., D.J. Callans, and F.E. Marchlinski, *Characterization of endocardial electrophysiological substrate in patients with nonischemic cardiomyopathy and monomorphic ventricular tachycardia.* Circulation, 2003. **108**(6): p. 704-10.

[46] Soejima, K., et al., *Endocardial and epicardial radiofrequency ablation of ventricular tachycardia associated with dilated cardiomyopathy: the importance of low-voltage scars.* J Am Coll Cardiol, 2004. **43**(10): p. 1834-42.

[47] de Bakker, J.M., et al., *Fractionated electrograms in dilated cardiomyopathy: origin and relation to abnormal conduction.* J Am Coll Cardiol, 1996. **27**(5): p. 1071-8.

[48] Nazarian, S., et al., *Magnetic resonance assessment of the substrate for inducible ventricular tachycardia in*

nonischemic cardiomyopathy. Circulation, 2005. **112**(18): p. 2821-5.

[49] Assomull, R.G., et al., *Cardiovascular magnetic resonance, fibrosis, and prognosis in dilated cardiomyopathy.* J Am Coll Cardiol, 2006. **48**(10): p. 1977-85.

[50] Bogun, F.M., et al., *Delayed-enhanced magnetic resonance imaging in nonischemic cardiomyopathy: utility for identifying the ventricular arrhythmia substrate.* J Am Coll Cardiol, 2009. **53**(13): p. 1138-45.

[51] Oloriz, T., et al., *Catheter ablation of ventricular arrhythmia in nonischemic cardiomyopathy: anteroseptal versus inferolateral scar sub-types.* Circ Arrhythm Electrophysiol, 2014. **7**(3): p. 414-23.

[52] Zeppenfeld, K., *Ventricular Tachycardia Ablation in Nonischemic Cardiomyopathy.* JACC Clin Electrophysiol, 2018. **4**(9): p. 1123-1140.

[53] Valles, E., V. Bazan, and F.E. Marchlinski, *ECG criteria to identify epicardial ventricular tachycardia in nonischemic cardiomyopathy.* Circ Arrhythm Electrophysiol, 2010. **3**(1): p. 63-71.

[54] Daniels, D.V., et al., *Idiopathic epicardial left ventricular tachycardia originating remote from the sinus of Valsalva: electrophysiological characteristics, catheter ablation, and identification from the 12-lead electrocardiogram.* Circulation, 2006. **113**(13): p. 1659-66.

[55] Hutchinson, M.D., et al., *Endocardial unipolar voltage mapping to detect epicardial ventricular tachycardia substrate in patients with nonischemic left ventricular cardiomyopathy.* Circ Arrhythm Electrophysiol, 2011. **4**(1): p. 49-55.

[56] Polin, G.M., et al., *Endocardial unipolar voltage mapping to identify epicardial substrate in arrhythmogenic right ventricular cardiomyopathy/ dysplasia.* Heart Rhythm, 2011. **8**(1): p. 76-83.

[57] Bala, R., et al., *Assessing epicardial substrate using intracardiac echocardiography during VT ablation.* Circ Arrhythm Electrophysiol, 2011. **4**(5): p. 667-73.

[58] Kumar, S., et al., *"Needle-in-needle" epicardial access: Preliminary observations with a modified technique for facilitating epicardial interventional procedures.* Heart Rhythm, 2015. **12**(7): p. 1691-7.

[59] Ludwig, D.R., et al., *A novel toolkit to improve percutaneous subxiphoid needle access to the healthy pericardial sac.* J Cardiovasc Electrophysiol, 2015. **26**(5): p. 576-80.

[60] Duvernoy, O., et al., *Pericardial effusion and pericardial compartments after open heart surgery. An analysis by computed tomography and echocardiography.* Acta Radiol, 1990. **31**(1): p. 41-6.

[61] Gale, M.E., M.G. Kiwak, and D.R. Gale, *Pericardial fluid distribution: CT analysis.* Radiology, 1987. **162**(1 Pt 1): p. 171-4.

[62] Keramati, A.R., et al., *Anterior pericardial access to facilitate electrophysiology study and catheter ablation of ventricular arrhythmias: A single tertiary center experience.* J Cardiovasc Electrophysiol, 2017. **28**(10): p. 1189-1195.

[63] Greenbaum, A.B., et al., *Intentional Right Atrial Exit and Carbon Dioxide Insufflation to Facilitate Subxiphoid Needle Entry Into the Empty Pericardial Space: First Human Experience.* JACC Clin Electrophysiol, 2015. **1**(5): p. 434-441.

[64] Long, D.Y., et al., *Pericardial access via wire-guided puncture without contrast:*

The feasibility and safety of a modified approach. J Cardiovasc Electrophysiol, 2020. **31**(1): p. 30-37.

[65] Silberbauer, J., et al., *Coronary Vein Exit and Carbon Dioxide Insufflation to Facilitate Subxiphoid Epicardial Access for Ventricular Mapping and Ablation: First Experience.* JACC Clin Electrophysiol, 2017. **3**(5): p. 514-521.

[66] Soejima, K., et al., *Subxiphoid surgical approach for epicardial catheter-based mapping and ablation in patients with prior cardiac surgery or difficult pericardial access.* Circulation, 2004. **110**(10): p. 1197-201.

[67] Koruth, J.S., et al., *Unusual complications of percutaneous epicardial access and epicardial mapping and ablation of cardiac arrhythmias.* Circ Arrhythm Electrophysiol, 2011. **4**(6): p. 882-8.

[68] Sosa, E. and M. Scanavacca, *Epicardial mapping and ablation techniques to control ventricular tachycardia.* J Cardiovasc Electrophysiol, 2005. **16**(4): p. 449-52.

[69] Bai, R., et al., *Phrenic nerve injury after catheter ablation: should we worry about this complication?* J Cardiovasc Electrophysiol, 2006. **17**(9): p. 944-8.

[70] Roberts-Thomson, K.C., et al., *Coronary artery injury due to catheter ablation in adults: presentations and outcomes.* Circulation, 2009. **120**(15): p. 1465-73.

[71] Steffel, J., et al., *2021 European Heart Rhythm Association Practical Guide on the Use of Non-Vitamin K Antagonist Oral Anticoagulants in Patients with Atrial Fibrillation.* Europace, 2021.